futures

social policy: welfare, power and diversity

series editor: john clarke

This book is part of a series produced in association with The Open University. The complete list of books in the series is as follows:

Embodying the Social: Constructions of Difference, edited by Esther Saraga

Forming Nation, Framing Welfare, edited by Gail Lewis

Welfare: Needs, Rights and Risks, edited by Mary Langan

Unsettling Welfare: The Reconstruction of Social Policy, edited by Gordon Hughes and Gail Lewis

Imagining Welfare Futures, edited by Gordon Hughes

The books form part of the Open University course D218 *Social Policy: Welfare, Power and Diversity*. Details of this and other Open University courses can be obtained from the Course Reservations Centre, PO Box 724, The Open University, Milton Keynes MK7 6ZS, United Kingdom: tel. (00 44) (0)1908 653231.

For availability of other course components, contact Open University Worldwide Ltd, The Berrill Building, Walton Hall, Milton Keynes MK7 6AA, United Kingdom: tel. (00 44) (0)1908 858585, fax (00 44) (0)1908 858787, e-mail ouwenq@open.ac.uk.

Alternatively, much useful course information can be obtained from the Open University's website http://www.open.ac.uk.

Cover: Photograph by Gary Kirkham

imagining
welfare
futures

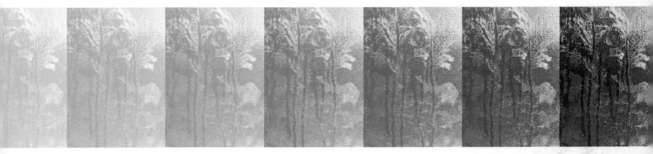

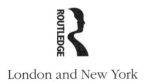

London and New York

in association with

The Open
University

edited
by
gordon
hughes

First published 1998 by Routledge
11 New Fetter Lane, London EC4P 4EE

Simultaneously published in the USA and Canada
by Routledge
29 West 35th Street, New York, NY 10001

BWC

Edited, designed and typeset by The Open University
Printed and bound by Scotprint Ltd, Musselburgh, Scotland

British Library Cataloguing in Publication Data
A catalogue record for this book is available from The British Library

Library of Congress Cataloguing in Publication Data
A catalogue record for this book has been requested

ISBN 0-415-18135-6 (hbk)
ISBN 0-415-18136-4 (pbk)

1.1

Contents

Preface

Imagining Welfare Futures is the final book in a new series of five introductory social policy texts published by Routledge in association with The Open University. The series, called *Social Policy: Welfare, Power and Diversity*, examines central issues in the study of how social welfare is organized in the UK today. The series is designed to provide a social scientific understanding of the complex and fascinating issues of social welfare in contemporary society. It specifically examines the key issues arising from questions concerning the changing nature of the welfare state and social policy in the UK, giving particular emphasis to the processes of social differentiation and their implications for social welfare. The series also emphasizes the ways in which social problems and solutions to them have been socially constructed and are subject to historical change. More generally, the books use social scientific theories and research studies together with, and in contrast to, other forms of 'knowing' about social welfare and social issues (such as common sense). This is done in order to raise key questions about how society 'works', how social change occurs, and how social order is maintained.

The five books form the core components of an Open University course which shares the title of this series. The first book, *Embodying the Social*, examines the central issue of how patterns of social difference are socially constructed. It traces the implications of such constructions for social policy – for example, the effects of shifting conceptions of disability – and examines their contested character. In exploring these concerns, this first book begins to establish the central focus of the course and series on *diversity*, the formations of *social difference*, and *power*, in particular the power to define our understanding of such differences.

The second book, *Forming Nation, Framing Welfare*, addresses the relationships between nation, state and social welfare by tracing the historical conflicts and constructions that have shaped our modern conceptions of national belonging and welfare rights and duties. The book explores the making of the nation – the inclusions and exclusions of different social groups – and the role of social policy in that process.

The third book, *Welfare: Needs, Rights and Risks*, focuses on a rather different issue, namely the questions of who gets welfare and under what conditions. This book examines how categories of need, desert, risk and rights play a central role in constructing access to welfare, particularly in circumstances where arguments over rationing, priority setting and limited resources are central to the forming of social policies.

The fourth book, *Unsettling Welfare*, deals with the rise and fall of the welfare state in the UK, and traces the ways in which the relationship between social welfare and the state has been reconstructed at the turn of the twentieth century. In particular, it focuses on the consequences of the break-up of the political, economic and social settlements that had sustained the 'old' welfare state in the thirty years after the Second World War.

This fifth and final book, *Imagining Welfare Futures*, looks at the prospects for the further remaking of social welfare around the focal points of citizenship, community and consumerism.

Because these books are integral elements of an Open University course, they are designed in distinctive ways in order to contribute to the process of student learning. Each book is constructed as an interactive teaching text, and this has implications for how the book can be read. The chapters form a planned sequence, so that each chapter builds on its predecessors and each concludes with a set of suggestions for further reading in relation to its core topics. The books are also organized around a series of learning processes:

- *Activities*: highlighted in colour, these are exercises which invite you to take an active part in working on the text and are intended to test your understanding and develop reflective analysis.

- *Comments*: these provide feedback from the chapter's author(s) on the activities and enable you to compare your responses with the thoughts of the author(s).

- *Shorter questions*: again highlighted in colour, these are designed to encourage you to pause and reflect on what you have just read.

- *Key words*: these are concepts or terms that play a central role in each chapter and in the course's approach to studying social policy; they are highlighted in colour in the text and in the margins.

While each book in the series is self-contained, there are also references backwards and forwards to the other books. Readers who wish to use the series as the basis for a systematic introduction to studying social policy should note that the references to chapters in other books of the series appear in bold type. The objective of this approach to presenting the material is to enable readers to grasp and reflect on the central themes, issues and arguments not only of each chapter, but also of each book and the series as a whole.

The production of this book and the others that make up the series draws on the expertise of a whole range of people beyond its editors and authors. Each book reflects the combined efforts of an Open University course team: the 'collective teacher' at the heart of the Open University's educational system. Each chapter in these books has been through a process of drafts and comments to refine both its content and its approach to teaching. This process of development leaves us indebted to our consultant authors, our panel of tutor advisers and our course assessor. It also brings together and benefits from a range of other skills – of our secretarial staff, editors, designers, librarians – to translate the ideas into the finished product. All of these activities are held together by the course manager, who ensures that all these component parts and people fit together successfully. Our thanks to them all.

John Clarke

Introduction

**by John Clarke, Gordon Hughes, Gail Lewis
and Gerry Mooney**

The meaning of the welfare state

At the turn of the twentieth century, there are problems about how to define the welfare state in the face of changing approaches to providing and delivering social welfare (**Hughes and Lewis, 1998**). The changes to which the welfare states in the UK and elsewhere have been subjected through the last twenty years of the century have made it more difficult to identify something distinctively marked out as a welfare state (Esping-Anderson, 1996). For example, there are problems about whether one takes the welfare state to refer to the services produced, provided and delivered by public agencies (Clarke, 1996), or whether we should use the term to include those benefits and services purchased by public resources but which may be provided by commercial or voluntary bodies.

Despite the significance of these definitional issues, the changes to social welfare also raise other, equally important questions. In particular, they have made visible a series of questions about *what the welfare state means*. The shifting arrangements of social welfare make it necessary to think about what the welfare state has symbolized in the past – what it used to stand for – and what the emerging new arrangements of social welfare might symbolize in their turn. Our interest here is in the way the idea of the welfare state has functioned symbolically as a representation of a set of relationships: relationships that link the state, social welfare and the people. It will be clear that we need to distinguish 'welfare' and 'the state' in talking about the symbolism of the welfare state. For most of the twentieth century, and certainly in the centuries preceding it, the terms 'welfare' and 'the state' did not fit naturally or comfortably together. Only in the years between 1945 and 1980 was there a strong connection between the two terms, such that 'the welfare state' became a commonplace phrase in political and public language. Its establishment as a term of public reference made it central to the conflicts of party politics in the second half of the twentieth century. It has played a role as a totem of political virility (the commitment to reform or even abolish the welfare state); of traditional loyalties (the commitment to keep the welfare state); and of pragmatic adaptation (the commitment to modernize the welfare state). In all of these – and many other variants – the welfare state has stood for something more than a specific set of policies, benefits or services. It has meant something more than just a set of organizations, agencies and workers. The phrase 'the welfare state' has implied something about the relationships between the people, their well-being and the state.

So, what did the welfare state mean in the post-war period? We need to be careful here, as it is rare for any social institution or practice to have just one uncontested meaning. With this in mind, though, it is possible to suggest some of the *dominant meanings* associated with the welfare state in public and political culture in the UK. The welfare state seemed to represent or stand for a number of integrative processes in British society: promoting *social* assistance and social security, through *collective* provision and *national* insurance and, possibly, even redressing *social* inequalities (Clarke *et al.*, 1987, pp.89–99). The meanings of the welfare state were those of social or collective integration, dealing in collective obligations to make provision for need, distress and disease, as well as making collective investments in the nation's future through child welfare, schooling, etc. Let us examine these images a little further. There is a narrative or storyline that underpins this dominant imagery of the welfare state:

- The people (the British public), having endured years of hardship, uncertainty and insecurity, had the need, wish or will to free themselves from such circumstances.

- The machinery through which this could be most effectively done was the state, which possessed the national scope, the expertise and the reliability to promote social welfare. Other agencies or mechanisms were, by contrast, partial, local, flawed or unreliable.

- The state thus came to embody the collective will to 'do something about' the Five Giants identified by William Beveridge in 1943 (Idleness, Ignorance, Want, Squalor and Disease).

- The state would therefore promote social welfare (security, assistance, etc.) in order to meet its obligations to the British people.

- Citizens would be enabled by social provision to be free of insecurity *and* the fear of insecurity. They would, as a result, be able to lead useful, productive and fulfilled lives.

Unlike more recent political conceptions of the failings of the welfare state, this 'founding' imagery of the 1940s and 1950s treated the sets of relationships between social welfare, the state and the people as both integrated and integrative. It was an image of how the welfare state would promote or enhance social integration, since all the people would be citizens whose social participation would be underpinned by these processes. These were the dominant, and mostly positive, images of the relationship between people, state and welfare associated with the post-war welfare state. There were other images and other attempts to portray those relationships. Some identified the welfare state as too much 'interference', as 'undermining' the British people and their way of life; or as a mere sop that propped up an ailing and dangerous capitalist system by making it look more pleasant (Clarke *et al.*, 1987, pp.85–126). Despite such conflicting perspectives, the post-war decades were dominated by the integrative imagery of 'social citizenship' associated with the Beveridge-based welfare state (Marshall, 1962).

These questions of what the welfare state stood for are only partly a matter of ideas. They are also about the ways in which such ideas were embodied in institutional arrangements and lived or experienced in practice. We might therefore talk about how the welfare state stood for or symbolized a particular view of the people (who the 'we' of the nation were); what 'our' relationship to the state was (how 'our' needs were to be served) and what our historical trajectory was (from the bleak depression years to a prospect of social improvement). But it is also important to pay attention to how these images were given life in practice in the institutional processes that made up the welfare state. Such processes were the practical connections that linked the people, social welfare and the state at an everyday level. Examples of such 'everyday' processes and practices might have included:

- being taken to school
- visiting a GP
- waiting in a social security office
- getting school milk
- attending a child welfare clinic
- being transported by ambulance
- having housing repairs done by council maintenance teams
- receiving 'meals on wheels'.

ACTIVITY

Think about an experience that defines or symbolizes the welfare state for you. What sorts of relationships did it embody? Were they positive or negative ones?

The multiple policies, practices and relationships that made up the welfare state carried sets of images about the people and their place in relation to the state. Some of these images involved messages about who 'the people' were: who counted as part of the people and who did not; how they should behave as part of the people; what they had in common and what set them apart from others. Some of these images involved messages about what 'welfare' meant: what sorts of misfortune, inequality or conditions could be a focus of public action; what problems could be addressed; what claims could be legitimately made on public institutions. Finally, some of these images of the welfare state carried messages about the role, purpose and character of the state itself: what should the state do; how far should it involve itself in what had been thought of as private matters; did the state act to enable, protect or control its citizens; how far should it enforce forms of welfare on people 'for their own good'; should the state provide 'universally' or 'selectively', and what sort of selectivity should there be? The idea of the welfare state embodied these sorts of images and the complex messages that they carry (see Figure 1). Our interactions with the welfare state engaged us in bits of these images: could we prove we were part of 'the people'; could we demonstrate that our needs were legitimate; could we accept others acting 'in our best interests'?

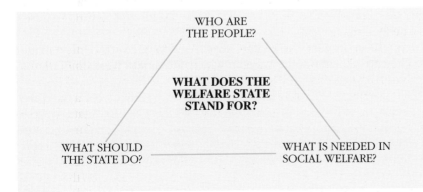

Figure 1

It is clear that these sets of meanings about the welfare state had become relatively established and institutionalized between the 1940s and 1970s, but subsequently became destabilized in the 1980s and 1990s. The result was to bring tensions and conflicts about the *meanings* of 'the people', 'welfare' and 'the state' into public view again. Before we look further at this re-opening of the conflicts over these ideas, it is worth stepping back a little to think about this approach to discussing the welfare state.

Representing the people

The discussion so far reflects a widespread interest within the social sciences in the production and circulation of meaning as a central feature of social organization. It is in this sense that we have been asking what the welfare state means. Actions, processes and institutions all carry meanings. At the most minimal level, such meanings are what enable us to go about our interactions in the expectation that others will understand us. If every time we spoke we had to pause to define each word we used, social life might be a lot slower and less smooth. However, as we have seen in relation to the imagery of the welfare state, meanings are neither simple nor uncontested. Because meanings affect how people act, they are the focus for conflicting attempts to make meaning. For example, those seeking to restructure the welfare state in the 1980s and 1990s expended considerable energy on trying to change the dominant imagery or meaning of the welfare state, constructing an alternative image of the welfare state as costly, intrusive, inefficient and damaging to the interests of the British people (**Lewis, 1998a**). The analytic concern with meaning and processes of social construction is one that has become increasingly significant in social sciences in the 1980s and 1990s (see, for example, Burr, 1995; **Clarke and Cochrane, 1998**). Here, though, we want to focus on a rather more specific set of issues: ones which centre on the process of *representation*. We have already made extensive use of terms like 'symbolize' and 'stand for'. Working out what the welfare state means involves treating it as 'standing for' or 'representing' a set of ideas, images or beliefs. Representation refers to the processes by which the social world is understood or made sense of by members of a society. The social world is represented to us through sets of knowledges, 'mental maps' or images that define us and our place in that world. Thus, the welfare state 'represented' a particular set of views about the nature of social welfare, the role and character of the state, and the social composition, needs and wishes of the 'British people'. Representation refers to a process through which meanings are constructed. In this sense it is rather different from its more technical usage in politics and public administration, where it is used to talk about how representatives are selected or chosen to express the views of the people (as in the Representation of the People Acts that govern the electoral process in the UK).

Our use of representation is a more social – and social constructionist – one which is concerned with the production and solidification of meaning. This idea of actions, people or institutions 'standing for' or 'representing' understandings of social relationships is something that has been developed very clearly in the study of traditions. Most of us can understand that the monarchy both refers to a particular family and 'stands for' a set of understandings of relationships between the British people, the Crown and the government. But the processes by which the monarchy acquires these meanings are not natural or inevitable; they are the result of struggles to make the monarchy mean these things (and not others). It is for these reasons that some historians have referred to 'the invention of tradition' (Hobsbawm and Ranger, 1983; Williams, 1985). For the purpose of this book, then, we are concerned with the ways in which the welfare state can *both* refer to a particular configuration of agencies, policies and practices *and* represent a set of understandings about the state, welfare and the people.

In many respects our concerns here are ones that have traditionally been associated with concepts of ideology and ideological struggle (Donald and Hall, 1986). Theories of ideology have tended to treat the issue of representation in one of two ways. The first, more instrumental, conception has seen ideologies as representing the interests of specific classes or social groups. Ideologies support, sustain or legitimate those interests. Here ideologies represent social groups rather in the way that MPs are supposed to represent the electorate – they 'stand for' them in a rather narrow and instrumental way. They 'transmit' the interests of those whom they represent. One of the classic statements of this view is Marx and Engels's claim in *The German Ideology* (written in 1846) that: 'the ideas of the ruling class are in every epoch the ruling ideas … The ruling ideas are nothing more than the ideal expression of the dominant material relationships grasped as ideas' (Marx and Engels, 1970, p.64). Although Marx and Engels elaborated this view of ideology in relation to dominant and subordinate social classes, other social scientists have used similarly instrumental conceptions of ideology to talk about a range of other social divisions and the ideas that have been used to sustain them (for example in analyses of sexism, racism or ageism).

An alternative approach to ideology was developed out of criticisms of the narrow instrumentalism of this view of one class having the 'ruling ideas'. This alternative sees social struggles as being conducted *through* ideology – in conflicts over meaning. This second approach has sometimes been described as a 'theory of articulation' (Slack, 1996). This phrase draws on the two meanings of the verb 'to articulate'. One meaning is that of expressing an idea or point of view, as in 'she tried to articulate the meaning of ideology in her own words'. The second meaning is that of connecting or creating a link or hinge between two or more things: for example, the elbow articulates the upper and lower arm. This approach to ideology uses the two meanings to treat ideologies as expressing or formulating meanings by connecting ideas to other ideas in chains of reasoning. Thus, the idea of 'freedom' is both highly valued and ambiguous. It plays a central role in political struggles because of the value it carries but also because it can be made to mean different things (such as the freedom to choose or freedom from want) by being connected to – or articulated with – other terms and ideas.

This approach opens up a rather more complicated view of ideological conflict. The simplest view is that different ideologies 'own' different words, exemplified in the view that an individualist ideology is centred on the word 'freedom', while a socialist ideology is centred on the word 'equality'. A theory of articulation, however, allows us to see how both individualist and socialist ideologies may use the word 'freedom' but will try to make it mean different things. Each ideology inflects or articulates 'freedom' in a different way. In the course of this book, we will see both of these processes in action. So, at some points, the identity of 'being a consumer' of social welfare is *opposed to* the identity of 'being a citizen' of a welfare state. It implies different positions and relationships. However, at other points, we will find attempts to define the character of 'citizenship' as meaning 'being a consumer' (as in the Citizen's Charter of the 1990s). This involved the attempt to inflect or articulate 'citizen' in a particular way: one which moved its meaning away from older social democratic views of citizenship rights.

This emphasis on articulation as the key process in ideological conflict has drawn heavily on the ideas of the Italian Marxist Antonio Gramsci (1971) and has been developed in contemporary social and political analysis in the work of Stuart Hall in particular (Hall, 1996). Both Hall and Gramsci placed special emphasis on the contested meanings of 'nation' and 'the people' as focal points of ideological conflict. Defining the boundary and character of the nation and defining the social composition, cultural traditions or 'way of life' of the people have been significant issues in the development of social welfare in the UK (**Lewis, 1998c**). Statements about action to be taken 'in the national interest' always raise questions about whose interests are being spoken for in this way (and whose are not) and how they come to be seen as national, rather than specific or partisan concerns. Ideological articulations of 'differences' between the English or British and others (foreigners, aliens, other 'races') have helped to define both the purpose and limits of welfare citizenship (**Morris, 1998**). Some writers have ascribed the term the 'national popular' to this field of constructions of the nation and the people, a term which indicates how closely enmeshed are images of nation and people (Forgacs, 1993). It is a term that will be used in later chapters of this book as they explore ways in which the relationships between the people and the nation state are being reimagined and represented.

This view of ideology directs us towards an understanding that the *process of representation* always involves a double movement. First, there are always multiple meanings available for any particular term or idea: thus, the 'British people' can be construed or defined in a number of different ways, with different social implications and more or less exclusive definitions of its 'membership'. But second, there are also continuing struggles over which of these possibilities becomes the dominant or (ideally) taken-for-granted and unquestioned meaning. Think, for example, of the way in which the phrase 'black British' disrupted one almost unquestioned assumption about the equivalence of 'the British people' and 'white people' (**Lewis, 1998b**). This book does not intend to explore all aspects of conflicts around the 'national popular' in the UK at the end of the twentieth century. There is a whole range of contested meanings and images that have addressed the form and limits of the 'nation'. For instance, changing political relationships with Europe have led to fierce conflicts about the meanings of 'Britishness' and 'Englishness'. Similarly, conflicts over national identity and political institutions have surrounded issues of independence, devolution and unification within and around the UK in ways that demonstrate the contested boundaries of 'nations'. Equally, there have been recurrent conflicts over the assumed social composition of 'the people'. Some of these have been about gender and sexuality; some about 'race', ethnicity and disability; some have been about age and the assumed dependency of the old and the young; while others have been about the existence of an 'excluded underclass' or the status of 'genuine' refugees. All of them concern who gets to be included in 'the people', and on what terms. Here, though, our focus of attention is rather more specific. We are concerned with the images through which the relationships between the people, the state and social welfare are being represented. The assumptions and conditions that sustained a post-war social democratic or 'Beveridgean' image of 'the public' and the welfare state had been dismantled by the 1990s. This book addresses the question of what might replace that imagery.

This focus of attention raises one other significant issue about ideology or the contested processes of social construction. These processes are not just about ideas: 'articulation' is not simply moving words around so that they mean something different. They are also processes through which identifications and attachments can be created – the symbolic means through which 'we' can recognize ourselves and see where 'we belong'. By implication, they are simultaneously processes of rejection, detachment and non-recognition. They position 'others' who do not or cannot belong and who are not spoken for in the construction of this particular 'we'. This aspect of articulation (or social construction) means giving attention to affective or non-rational dimensions of meaning as well as the more instrumental or rational views about social interests and ideology. The processes of identification ('I am part of this') and attachment ('I belong here – I am represented in this institution') are complex ones. They are extremely solid and durable, bound up in deeply sedimented ideas about the nation, its social institutions, its way of life and its traditions. They are also extremely fluid and delicate at both the collective and individual level. The ways of life change, and so do the social and political institutions in which 'we' are supposed to find ourselves represented. Sometimes 'we' believe that the institutions 'need to change' to catch up with who and where 'we' are. For example, the 1990s were marked by a variety of demands that social and political institutions should 'modernize' themselves. The monarchy, the judiciary, the BBC and the armed forces all encountered demands that they should be less 'out of touch' and more 'representative' of a modern United Kingdom.

In trying to analyse the contested and problematic constructions of the people, state and social welfare, we have found it useful to draw on a concept developed by Raymond Williams when he was analysing literary culture in his book *The Long Revolution* (1965). Williams used the phrase 'a structure of feeling' as a way of defining the cluster of dominant images, meanings and sentiments in a specific culture. Most cultural analysts have avoided the phrase because of its ambiguous, if not paradoxical, character: the words 'structure' and 'feeling' do not sit obviously or comfortably together. Nevertheless, we have found it useful precisely because it combines these two aspects. Williams himself approaches the idea by pointing out how 'between generations' or between people who are 'part of a community' and 'outsiders' there are disjunctures of meaning and understanding in which central, but usually unstated, cultural assumptions become exposed. This bears some similarity to social science approaches that attempt to uncover the 'common-sense' or 'taken-for-granted' elements of social life (**Clarke and Cochrane, 1998**). Williams (1965, p.65) then goes on to discuss what is revealed in such moments: 'The term I would suggest to describe it is *structure of feeling*: it is as firm and definite as "structure" suggests, yet it operates in the most delicate and least tangible parts of our activity. In one sense, this structure of feeling is the culture of a period.'

Williams's focus of attention is the expression of such 'structures of feeling' in literary and artistic cultural forms: novels, plays, paintings, and so on. Our concern is with social and political forms: the images and representations that express or articulate a 'structure of feeling' about how the people, state and social welfare are interconnected. The concept of a 'structure of feeling' is important for us because it draws attention to the problem of analysing these images and representations. They are both 'firm and definite' and delicate, needing to be teased out and explored with care. In the three main chapters of the book, we will be exploring three different 'structures of feeling': three ways of making sense of the relationships that link people, the state and social welfare. They are 'definite': they are organized around three core images of the people as consumers, communities and citizens. But they are also delicate and intangible, in part because they are not clear, unequivocal statements or manifestos, but also because they offer points of identification, attachment or recognition in which we are invited to glimpse ourselves.

There are many other arguments (and disputes) in the study of ideologies and discourses, but they are not central to our purposes here. In developing our discussion of different welfare futures in the remainder of this book, we want to be clear that we are approaching it with the following analytical perspective in mind:

- That we are dealing with representations of 'imagined or imaginary relations', with a particular focus on the imaginary relations that connect 'the people', 'the state' and 'social welfare'.

- That we are dealing with attempts to connect meanings with political strategies or directions. For example, different strategies may want to use the word 'citizen' (because of its positive social resonances) but will try to make it mean something different within their chains of representations.

- That we will be addressing not just 'ideas' but ideologies (or discourses) that are embedded in social processes and practices in ways that give them a sense of depth and density that cannot be claimed by 'abstract ideas' alone. For example, the word 'community' is suffused with the sense that many people live in, believe they live in (that is, represent themselves as living in), or wish they lived in, a 'community'.

- That we will be dealing with 'contested' strategies that have attempted to define the future imaginary relationships that link the people, the state and social welfare – to establish themselves as the new 'taken-for-granted' representations of how it is and should be.

The assault on 'the public'

With these ideas in mind, we can return to the changing fortunes of the UK welfare state between 1945 and 2000 and ask what has happened to what the welfare state stands for. The crisis of the welfare state has been widely discussed. It has been explained in relation to the economy, changing political regimes, declining public legitimacy, the loss of faith in the state as a solution to social problems, and so on. Rather less attention has been given to the changing imaginary relationships of people, state and social welfare associated with the crisis of the welfare state. Although this crisis is conventionally discussed in terms of the economic dislocations and changes of the mid 1970s onwards and the assault by the New Right on the old 'social democratic' political consensus about the role of the welfare state, there were significant problems associated with the imaginary relations of the old welfare state that contributed to the sense of crisis (**Hughes, 1998**). These mark the limits and limitations of the imaginary relationships of the post-war welfare state. New social movements and new social subjects (**Lewis, 1998a**; Williams, 1994 and 1996) challenged the comfortable imaginary relationship of people, state and social welfare. In particular, they challenged:

- the imagery of the people as (white) 'British citizens', familialized in a conventional division of labour between male 'breadwinners' and women-as-wives-and-mothers;
- the imagery of the state as a neutral instrument of social improvement;
- the imagery of social welfare as universal, benevolent and enabling.

New social movements articulated around struggles over 'race', gender, sexuality and disability attacked the partial and paternalistic character of this social democratic imagery of 'the people'. They did so by demonstrating the structured nature of inclusions and exclusions of membership in the nation and the hierarchical positioning of different sorts of membership. They challenged assumptions about the 'dependency' or 'problem status' attributed to those who were not white, able-bodied males. They pointed to the role of the state in reproducing rather than remedying some forms of inequality and discrimination – both in its welfare policies and in its employment practices. Finally, they challenged conceptions of welfare as benevolent and progressive by identifying the often oppressive and discriminatory nature of bureaucratic and professional processes. These assaults on the old welfare state also challenged the limits of what was understood to be 'social'. In the old social democratic conception, social inequality was primarily, if not exclusively, a question of class (understood in terms of inequalities of income and wealth). Other divisions and inequalities were rarely conceived of as social. 'Race', gender, disability, age and sexuality were all treated as naturally (biologically) occurring differences. Such differences might create 'special needs' for assistance, treatment or control, but they were not socially produced and so could not be redressed by social action.

Such challenges to the imaginary relations of the social democratic welfare state coexisted with other – and rather different – ideological assaults, in particular from the New Right and its influence on the Conservative governments of the 1980s and 1990s. The New Right was self-consciously opposed to the social democratic (or 'socialist', as they usually called it) settlements and their conceptions of state, people and social welfare. A central theme of their ideological politics was the dismantling or unlocking of the 'national popular' imagery of social democracy and the need to replace it with different representations of the British people. The welfare state had to be reformed (if not abolished) both for political and economic reasons, but also because it was the practical embodiment of these social democratic imaginary relations. There – in state schools, in council housing rentbooks, in NHS outpatient departments, and so on – were the interactions that reminded everybody, on an everyday basis, of the social democratic representations of people, state and social welfare.

The social democratic representation of citizenship was not just an idea but was lived and experienced (for good or ill) in those daily encounters.

This social democratic imagery thus constituted a particular 'structure of feeling'. It organized identities, positions and attachments around the idea of the welfare state. It drew on and reproduced a specific understanding of the people with assumptions about their social composition and ways of life. It represented their needs and problems as being addressed by the policies and institutions of the welfare state. 'The people' (and the national interest), social welfare and the state were united in this image of the welfare state. It embodied and expressed the collective provision needed to secure 'the public interest'. Images of the public were central to this social democratic structure of feeling. First, there were representations of people as 'the public' (collectively) and as 'members of the public' (individually). Second, there were notions of a 'public interest' in promoting social welfare, solving problems and bringing about social improvements that was expected to override or limit individual or sectional interests. Third, there was a sense that the pursuit of the public interest or the public good was best accomplished by public institutions and organizations (the state), because private organizations were motivated by other concerns (notably the search for profit). Fourth, such public institutions were represented as being staffed by 'public servants', motivated and controlled by an ethos or set of values that placed a priority on promoting 'the public interest' rather than selfish interest.

By the early 1990s most of the elements of this social democratic structure of feeling had been destabilized by a range of challenges, but especially by the New Right's hostility to all these images of 'the public' (Clarke and Newman, 1997). The New Right insisted that, in almost every respect, the public came a poor second to 'the private'. Private enterprise was more efficient and effective than public organizations. Private interests (in promoting one's own welfare) had been suppressed by the supposed 'public interest'. 'Public service' had been a disguise which concealed the real motives of venal or self-interested bureaucrats and professionals. The New Right championed a 'private' structure of feeling to replace the 'public' one of social democracy. In doing so, it articulated two different but essential senses of the term 'private'. First, there was the construction of private as referring to private *individuals and families*, who were understood as making choices for themselves about their own needs. Second, there was the construction of private as referring to 'the private sector' or 'the market' in contrast to 'the public sector' or 'the state'. The effect of the articulation of these different senses of 'private' was to construct a sequence of equivalences about private interests. The private interests of individuals (to get ahead, make choices, make money to meet their needs) were the same as the interests of private sector organizations (to compete successfully, be free of interference, make profits) which were, in turn, the same as the interests of the nation – 'UK plc' (to compete in the world economy; be free of red tape; be able to 'pay its way', and so on).

The 1980s and 1990s saw sustained attacks both on the structures and policies of the old welfare state and on the social democratic representations that were embodied in it. Their effect has been to dislocate the old imaginary relations of welfare, state and people. It is no longer possible to talk about an entity called 'the welfare state', since welfare and the state are, once again, no longer synonymous. The development of 'alternative providers' of social welfare, the development of more 'mixed economies' of welfare, the withdrawal of the state from some service provision, the growing emphasis on 'self-provisioning' or 'do it yourself' welfare all mean that the welfare state – as institution and as a representation – is not what it was. In the process, the New Right tried to redefine each of the three terms – welfare, the state and the people – as well as the relationships between them.

As we write this at the end of the 1990s, it is not clear what has replaced the old social democratic representations. It is clear, however, that they have been substantially unlocked or loosened, and they no longer exert the hold on British public discourse that they did in the high tide of 'welfarism'. In the following chapters we explore three possible ways of reimagining or reinventing the relationships between the people, welfare and the state. For convenience, we have treated them as if each centred around one particular representation – the people as consumers, the people as citizens, and the people as a community. In practice, of course, it is more complicated than this. When reading the following chapters, there are three issues to keep in mind about the ways in which these representations of imaginary relations are complicated.

First, each term involves a more complex set of representations, including conflicts over what the core term might mean – how it might be *articulated* to particular political strategies or directions. Thus, citizenship – although associated with the 'old social democratic' representations of people, state and welfare – has been 'reinvented' in a number of different ways.

Second, as part of wider ideological processes, none of these core terms is 'pure' or the property of one political position. Thus, those arguing for a view of state/welfare/people relationships to be understood and organized in terms of citizenship may nevertheless use the terms consumer or community as subordinate parts of their package of representations.

Third, we are describing ideological struggles that are *unfinished.* The three 'imaginary relations' discussed here are attempts to reinvent and reorganize the state, welfare and people relationships in new ways. By the time we have finished writing this, there may be other alternatives: new 'big ideas' may be presented for the future of welfare. Alternatively, one or more of those which we discuss may have dropped from sight. What we are sure about is that these attempts to reimagine the future of welfare will go on – and they will have to negotiate the basic terms of this issue in some form or another. They will have to offer representations of the imaginary relations of welfare, the state and the people.

References

Burr, V. (1995) *An Introduction to Social Constructionism*, London, Routledge.

Clarke, J. (1996) 'The problem of the state after the welfare state', in May, M., Brunsdon, E. and Craig, G. (eds) *Social Policy Review 8*, London, Social Policy Association.

Clarke, J. and Cochrane, A. (1998) 'The social construction of social problems', in Saraga (ed.) (1998).

Clarke, J., Cochrane, A. and Smart, C. (1987) *Ideologies of Welfare*, London, Routledge.

Clarke, J. and Newman, J. (1997) *The Managerial State: Power, Politics and Ideology in the Remaking of Social Welfare*, London, Sage.

Donald, J. and Hall, S. (eds) (1986) *Politics and Ideology*, Milton Keynes, Open University Press.

Esping-Anderson, G. (ed.) (1996) *Welfare States in Transition*, London, Sage.

Forgacs, D. (1993) 'National-popular: genealogy of a concept', in During, S. (ed.) *Cultural Studies Reader*, London, Routledge.

Gramsci, A. (1971) *Selections from the Prison Notebooks*, London, Lawrence and Wishart.

Hall, S. (1996) 'Gramsci's relevance to the study of ethnicity', in Morley and Chen (eds) (1996).

Hobsbawm, E. and Ranger, T. (eds) (1983) *The Invention of Tradition*, Cambridge, Cambridge University Press.

Hughes, G. (ed.) (1998) 'Picking over the remains: the welfare state settlements of the post-Second World War UK', in Hughes and Lewis (eds) (1998).

Hughes, G. and Lewis, G. (eds) (1998) *Unsettling Welfare: The Reconstruction of Social Policy*, London, Routledge in association with The Open University.

Lewis, G. (1998a) 'Coming apart at the seams: the crises of the welfare state', in Hughes and Lewis (eds) (1998).

Lewis, G. (1998b) 'Welfare and the social construction of "race"', in Saraga (ed.) (1998).

Lewis, G. (ed.) (1998c) *Forming Nation, Framing Welfare*, London, Routledge in association with The Open University.

Marshall, T.H. (1962) *Social Policy*, London, Hutchinson.

Marx, K. and Engels, F. (1970) *The German Ideology*, ed. with an introduction by C.J. Arthur, London, Lawrence and Wishart.

Morley, D. and Chen, K-H. (eds) (1996) *Stuart Hall: Critical Dialogues in Cultural Studies*, London, Routledge.

Morris, L. (1998) 'Legitimate membership of the welfare community', in Langan, M. (ed.) *Welfare: Needs, Rights and Risks*, London, Routledge in association with The Open University.

Saraga, E. (ed.) *Embodying the Social: Constructions of Difference*, London, Routledge in association with The Open University.

Slack, J. (1996) 'The theory and method of articulation in cultural studies', in Morley and Chen (eds) (1996).

Williams, G. (1985) *When Was Wales?*, London, Penguin.

Williams, F. (1994) 'Social relations, welfare and the post-Fordism debate', in Burrows, R. and Loader, B. (eds) *Towards a Post-Fordist Welfare State?*, London, Routledge.

Williams, F. (1996) 'Postmodernism, feminism and the question of difference', in Parton, N. (ed.) *Social Theory, Social Change and Social Work*, London, Routledge.

Williams, R. (1965) *The Long Revolution*, Harmondsworth, Penguin.

CHAPTER I

Consumerism

by John Clarke

Contents

1   Introduction

This chapter explores the figure of the consumer as one way of representing the relationship between members of society and the provision of social welfare. Unlike ideas of community and the citizen, this image is a relatively recent one in relation to social welfare. The first part of the chapter (sections 2 and 3) explores some of the reasons for the emergence of the consumer figure, particularly its place in the arguments about the relative advantages of markets and states as systems for distributing goods and services. It also examines the way in which practices of consuming goods and services provide a basis in everyday experience for the image of consumerism in social welfare.

The chapter goes on in section 4 to consider some of the changes that took place in the 1990s in the organization of welfare services which developed consumerist relationships between the state and members of the public. This leads to an examination of what sorts of consumers were created by these changes, since almost all commentators agree that the changes produced something other than the conventional consumer relationship of private market transactions. This second part of the chapter also looks at some evidence from research about how people go about acting as consumers in these new relationships with welfare services. This suggests that we need to think of consumers as *socially differentiated*.

The third part of the chapter (section 5) addresses a range of critical evaluations of these changes and the place of consumerist imagery in social welfare. These evaluations range from claims that such changes have not gone far enough, to arguments that consumerism is the wrong sort of relationship on which to base the organization of welfare services. The chapter concludes in section 6 by considering what sort of welfare futures might emerge if consumerism became the dominant form of relationship that structured the provision of welfare benefits and services.

2   Going to market

markets

The 1980s and 1990s were remarkable for the widespread assumptions that economies were the most important feature of societies and that markets were the best means of co-ordinating human activities. These assumptions were linked to a perception that processes of 'globalization' of production and distribution and increasing international competition were making national economies more vulnerable. These views underpinned growing political concern about the relationships between economies, markets and social life. Descriptions of national societies as corporate entities ('UK plc') were one indicator of these changes; another was the presumption that nations, corporations and individuals were all motivated by the same set of drives (entrepreneurial competitiveness) and would respond to the same 'sticks and carrots' (lower taxes, less regulation, greater freedom of choice, etc.). They would all, if set free from 'interference', pursue the same goals in dynamic and enterprising ways (see Keat and Abercrombie, 1991; du Gay, 1996). In the process, ideas of altruism, collectivism and mutuality were recurrently derided as concealing or distracting from the real human motivations of competitive and possessive individualism. At root, this view of 'economic man' saw the defining features of human behaviour as the wish to do better and the wish to own property.

As part of this process, contrasts were made between the 'market' and the 'state' as mechanisms for co-ordinating the distribution of goods and services to the members of society. Most of these contrasts were to the detriment of the 'state', which was almost uniformly regarded as less efficient and less effective, as well as more unnatural and distorting of human activity. It is important to note, before we go any further, that we are firmly within the realm of images and social constructions here, and I am using inverted commas around 'market' and 'state' as a way of reminding us that what are being discussed and compared are *ideas* of the market and state. This is sometimes visible in the style of argument in the extracts that follow, but it is important to keep it in mind throughout this section. So, what sort of contrasts were made?

ACTIVITY I.I

You should now read Extract 1.1 by Norman Barry. While you are doing so, you should try to make notes in relation to the following questions:

I   What advantages of the market are identified?

2   What failings of the state are identified?

3   What are the implications for the organization of social welfare?

The extract is mainly directed to the first two questions, so you are likely to have more difficulty with question 3.

Extract I.I Barry: 'Understanding the market'

One of the most striking features of the development of social science during the last decade has been the re-establishment of the intellectual respectability of the decentralized market exchange system as a social institution. There has been a growing recognition of both the efficiency and freedom-enhancing properties of market society. Many socialists now admit that planned, centralized economies have performed very badly in both these respects and are now anxious to incorporate at least some features of the market in their blueprints (redprints?) for the future …

What, then, lies behind the increased demands for 'privatization', a reduced role for the public sector and the 'rolling back of the state' that are heard from a wide variety of political sources in the contemporary world?

Perhaps the matter may be clarified by identifying three possible ways of organizing a society for the production of *wanted* goods and services: altruism, central command and the market. Altruism presupposes that individuals, without either the incentives of personal gain or fear of punishment, will satisfy the wants of others in a system of generalized reciprocity. It is now generally agreed that this places impossible burdens on a fragile human nature and on human knowledge. In a large society, even if people were uncommonly well-disposed towards each other, how could they *know* what others' wants were? In fact, altruism is only conceivable in very small communities where there is a broad agreement about ends and purposes. This leaves only central command and individual decision-making as serious alternatives. The critique of central command will emerge from a consideration of the market.

A market form of organization assumes that, from a *given* distribution of property rights and claims to natural resources (about which there can, of course, be much dispute) a predictable order will emerge from individual decisions. The market order is powered primarily by the price mechanism – which is no more than an indicator of the *scarcity* of resources in a community. Thus if there is a spontaneous demand for a commodity, or factor of production (labour, land or capital), its price will rise and therefore a signal is put out which brings forth extra supplies of the wanted good or factor of production. Without the guidance of price nobody would know what to do, and without the incentive to act, via profit, nothing would be produced.

What follows from this is that a decentralized exchange system, conducted within a general system of law (crime, contract and tort, etc.), requires very little in the way of centralized direction and control. A market is in essence a self-regulating, self-correcting system in which supply and demand and profit and loss are said to allocate resources more efficiently, and therefore 'solve' the perennial 'economic problem' of scarcity, better than any known alternative. Each participant in the process has to know only those economic facts that affect him personally since the market's signals, in F.A. von Hayek's words, 'enable individual producers to watch merely the movements of a few pointers, as an engineer might watch the hands of a few dials, in order to adjust their activities to changes of which they may never know more than is reflected in the prices movement' (Hayek, 1948, p.87).

This is a simple idea which tells us little about the structure of an advanced capitalist economy. But it is a very important concept because it shows how, in principle, the activities of disparate and decentralized individuals may be co-ordinated, as if, in Adam Smith's memorable phrase, by an 'Invisible Hand'. For the price system is constantly reflecting those changes in tastes, technology and availability of resources that characterize a complex society. Of course, it does not reflect these instantaneously, but its reactions to changes in these data are quicker than those of humanly devised institutions.

It would be inaccurate to describe all this as laissez-faire, a much abused term: a better phrase is Smith's 'the system of natural liberty'. By this he meant that through people's natural tendency to 'truck, barter and exchange' a movement to equilibrium operates, that is, a situation in which the *interdependent* parts of an economy cannot be rearranged to bring about an improved allocation of resources. In *The Wealth of Nations* (1776) he wrote: 'No regulation of commerce can increase the quantity of industry in any part of society beyond what its capital can maintain. It can only divert a part of it into a direction which it might otherwise not have gone' (Smith, 1976, p.453). Smith's implicit welfare judgement here is that governments are inevitably inferior to decentralized individuals in the production of wanted goods and services: 'I have never known much good done by those who affected to trade for the public good' (Smith, 1976, p.453). He said this not merely to doubt the automatic benevolence of governors (although he certainly did) but also to stress the fact that public beneficence always emerges as the *unintended consequence* of private, self-regarding action …

The movement towards a free and more competitive economy necessitates a sceptical attitude towards the state. The market theorist doubts that officials, elected or appointed, are motivated to act for the public good. He assumes they are no less immune to self-interest than familiar market transactors. Elected politicians are likely to provide policies favourable to politically significant interest groups while officials are motivated by non-pecuniary forms of aggrandizement, such as expansions of the size of their bureaux. The difficulty with a market society is that its benefits tend to be long-term and thinly spread while the advantages of political action, such as a state subsidy or an exemption from competition, are immediate to special interest groups. However, the sum of such privileges is damaging to the competitive market economy as a whole.

References

Hayek, F.A. (1948) *Individualism and Economic Order*, London, Routledge and Kegan Paul.

Smith, A. (1976) *An Enquiry into the Nature and Causes of the Wealth of Nations*, eds R.H. Campbell and A.S. Skinner, Oxford, Clarendon Press (first published 1776).

(Barry, 1991, pp.231–3)

COMMENT

The advantages of the market are claimed to be its responsiveness, its ability to co-ordinate a multiplicity of individual decisions, its capacity for driving out inefficient suppliers through competition, and its sponsoring of innovation and dynamism. By contrast, the state is seen as unresponsive, and bases decisions on inappropriate or inadequate information. The state is inefficient and its effects are anti-competitive.

The implications for social welfare are slightly more complicated. One implication is that the state should provide little or even no welfare benefits and services itself, precisely because it is inefficient. Individuals should make their own welfare decisions in a market context where they can choose between competing providers, who will be driven to provide better or cheaper services through competition.

■ ■ ■

It is important to take note of what these arguments address, because in the politics of welfare in the 1980s and 1990s they were often put forward together with other arguments about why state welfare provision was a bad thing. Here we are dealing with *neo-liberal* arguments which assume that individuals will wish to promote their own well-being. The central issue concerns the most efficient and effective means of providing such benefits and services, and the claim is that the market is better suited to promoting such efficiency and effectiveness than the state. This is not the same as arguments that the welfare state promoted dependency or demoralized the poor, or that it created social problems or undermined social authority. Such *neo-conservative* arguments concentrated on what we might call the moral, cultural or social effects of state action. Both neo-liberals and neo-conservatives argued for the state to reduce or withdraw from its welfare role, but for rather different reasons. They were often combined in New Right political ideology (Clarke, 1991).

3 Buying power: everyday consumers

In the previous section we examined relatively abstract ideas about the market. Though abstract, they clearly laid a foundation for public debates about providing social welfare. The ideas imply, rather than directly identify, the consumer role in market mechanisms, since part of the supposed dynamism and efficiency of market mechanisms results from placing the consumer at their centre (Larner, 1997). Consumers are economic actors who get to *choose*, and their choices are co-ordinated by the market in ways that squeeze out inefficient providers and reward efficient ones. Although these are rather dry and distant ideas of the

consumers

consumer, the *image* of the consumer also refers to our more mundane or common-sense knowledges about individuals, households and social behaviour. In the late twentieth century, we have become increasingly accustomed to meeting many of our everyday needs through the market-place (Gardner and Sheppard, 1989; Cahill, 1994). We now expect to have to purchase many of our basic needs: accommodation, food, clothes, heating, transport and the pleasures of free time (sports, entertainment, etc.). We understand the role of 'being a consumer'. We understand the idea of going shopping to meet our needs. We have experienced negotiating our wants against what the market-place can offer

cash nexus

through what social scientists call the cash nexus: the process of exchanging money for goods or services. Although *consuming* or consumption describes an activity in which we 'use up' something, the idea of 'being a consumer' is strongly linked to the *activity of purchasing* the object to be consumed – the point of exchange between buyer and seller (Clarke, 1991). For example, we have always 'consumed' food (in the sense of eating it), but it is only in the late twentieth century that we have become 'food consumers' in the sense of there being an elaborate and complex market in food supply (both from shops and restaurants) in which many people get to exercise some choices. In the following extract Judith Williamson addresses some issues about consumption – and the act of owning something that it implies – as a form of social power.

ACTIVITY 1.2

Now read Extract 1.2, which is from an article written by Judith Williamson in the 1980s. The article addresses some of the concerns of the Left about 'privatization' and 'consumerism' in Conservative welfare policies. What are Williamson's main points about the importance of power in relation to consumption?

Extract 1.2 Williamson: 'The politics of consumption'

The conscious, chosen meaning in most people's lives comes much more from what they consume than what they produce. Clothes, interiors, furniture, records, knick-knacks, all the things that we buy involve decisions and the exercise of our own judgement, choice, 'taste'. Obviously we don't choose what is available for us to choose between in the first place. Consuming seems to offer a certain scope for creativity, rather like a toy where all the parts are pre-chosen but the combinations are multiple. Consumerism is often represented as a supremely individualistic act – yet it is also very social: shopping is a socially endorsed event, a form of social cement. It makes you feel normal. Most people find it cheers them up – even window shopping. The extent to which shoplifting is done where there is no material need (most items stolen are incredibly trivial) reveals the extent to which people's wants and needs are *translated* into the form of consumption.

Buying and owning, in our society, offer a sense of control. If you pay for something you do tend to feel you control it; a belief borne out by people's eagerness to buy British Telecom shares regardless of the fact that they *already* owned BT. Yet the idea of having a stake in society or a tiny voting right in a public institution is not of itself reactionary, only the form it appears in. Although at present the left shies away from many issues of public ownership, surely the enormous rush of small-scale BT investors shows, not that everyone is a rabid 'Thatcherite', but that a great many 'ordinary' people do want 'a stake in this country' – something which they (like so many NHS patients) were evidently not made to *feel* they had when it was owned by the state.

Ownership is at present the *only* form of control legitimized in our culture. Any serious attempts at controlling products from the other side – as with the miners' demand to control the future of *their* product, coal (or the printing unions' attempts to control their product, newspaper articles, etc.) are not endorsed. Some parts of the left find these struggles less riveting than the struggles over meanings in street style. Yet underlying *both* struggles is the need for people to control their environment and produce their own communal identity; it is just that the former, if won, could actually fulfil that need while the latter ultimately never will. 'Progressive' socialists who argue that 'Thatcherism' has captured many popular needs are quite right – but while such needs are *captured* by this system they are precisely *not* fulfilled by it, in the way that they could be by a more daring socialism.

The point about consumerism is that people are getting something out of it – but something which the left must be able to offer *in a different form*. The current drift towards right-wing programmes on the left – e.g. the sale of council houses – because they are 'popular', ignores the possibility that many needs and ideals currently fulfilled by – to pursue this example – the ideology of home ownership, could be met in different ways. Some of the left seems now to have accepted the bourgeois equation of private ownership with freedom and the devolution of power – precisely the concepts behind Mrs Thatcher's election victories. It is as if the left can think of no other way to win than by imitating its enemies. The reason council tenants want to buy their houses is quite simple. They are not besotted with the idea of *ownership*; they are gripped by the need for *security*. The key emotions underpinning the dream of home ownership for most council tenants are the desires for control, autonomy and continuity. It should be possible for *public* housing to provide these by, for example, building into its principles the notion of the control of the individual tenant and in practice giving council tenants the feeling that their council flat or house *is* 'their' home.

(Williamson, 1987, pp.230–2)

COMMENT

Williamson constructs a complex argument about consumerism. She challenges the dismissive views of those of the traditional Left who fail to see how consumerism addresses people's needs for security and control in their lives. However, Williamson also suggests that consuming is not the only way in which such needs might be met. She insists that other ways of meeting aspirations and needs have to be developed because private ownership is a flawed and limited relationship. What is significant for us, though, is her consideration of why 'the consumer' is such a potent image. It carries social force because it links 'private' needs, aspirations, fears and dreams to a mechanism that promises to deal with them. Here we can see 'the consumer' as the central figure in a structure of feeling (see the Introduction to this book) that combines solidity (the act of buying, the fact of ownership) with more intangible sentiments and values (control, security, achievement).

control

structure of feeling

■ ■ ■

In Extract 1.2 Williamson refers to one of the first appearances of 'consumerism' in the Conservative government's welfare reforms of the 1980s: the 'right to buy' programme for council housing. This policy marked the start of a sustained challenge to the old user identities in the welfare state: 'tenant of the housing department', 'client of social services', 'doctor's patient', etc. During the 1980s and 1990s, all of these identities were reinvented in a more consumerist form.

To some extent this might have reflected the adaptation of welfare services to the growing centrality of consumerism in other areas of social life. As Dowding and Dunleavy (1996, p.40) suggest, 'the strong drift in modern capitalism is for consumers to demand private-sector point-of-service standards in all their dealings with formal organizations, a standard with which government enterprises find it very difficult to compete'. Such pressures were also politically focused around the consumer figure, primarily by the New Right, in claims that the exercise of consumer choice was the 'normal' way of life. Why shouldn't people choose schools, doctors, pensions, and so on in the same way that they choose food, clothes or cars? Keat *et al.* have suggested that the arguments around consumerism and social welfare have generally involved two related, but distinct, sets of propositions:

> 1 That the 'production' of such goods and services should be organized in ways that significantly mirror or parallel those involved in a free market economy, for example through the use of mechanisms enabling competition between rival producers, of contractually specified forms of exchange, and so on.

> 2 That the 'consumers' of these goods and services should enjoy the kind of relationship with their 'producers' that may be thought to obtain between actual consumers and producers in a free market economy – and hence, for example, that these goods and services should satisfy their consumers' preferences, be responsive to their demands, and so on.

> (Keat *et al.*, 1994, p.2)

There are important differences between these two propositions. The first concerns the construction of *market-like conditions*, stressing competition between providers or 'producers' as the basis for consumers to exercise choice. The second, by contrast, focuses on creating *relationships* that reflect or mimic desired features of consumerism, but do not necessarily involve markets. As we will see later, both of these approaches were pursued in relation to new forms of organizing social welfare in the late twentieth century. Both also bring with them particular sorts of problems. However, the consumer came to be represented as the most normal and most desirable role through which people's wants and needs could be met. Where the old state welfare systems had been organized around the principle of views being channelled through elected representatives, the dominant argument became that the provision of social welfare needed to approximate the conditions of the market through creating the possibility of choice. This distinction has been most clearly articulated in Hirschman's (1970) contrast between processes of 'voice' and 'exit', which are ways in which an organization's management might discover problems about its products or failings in its services:

> 1 Some customers stop buying the firm's products or some members leave the organization: this is the *exit option*. As a result, revenues drop, membership declines and management is impelled to search for ways and means to correct whatever faults have led to exit.

> 2 The firm's customers or the organization's members express their dissatisfaction directly to the management or to some other authority to which management is subordinate or through general protest addressed to anyone who cares to listen: this is the *voice option*. As a result, management once again engages in a search for the causes and possible cures of customers' and members' dissatisfaction.

> (Hirschman, 1970, p.4)

You will see that there are some links here with the two propositions outlined by Keat *et al.* For the 'exit' option to be effective, market-like conditions of *competing producers/providers* have to exist. Consumers need to be able to 'take their business elsewhere'. For the 'voice' option to be effective, a *relationship* has to exist in which the producer/provider wants to hear the consumer's voice in order to be responsive to their needs and views. Hirschman's distinction between 'voice' and 'exit' became a commonplace of discussions about the future of the welfare state during the late 1980s and 1990s because it provided a clear distinction between two contending views of, and processes for, representing the wishes of service users.

4 Constructing the consumer

In this second part of the chapter we will examine some of the changes in the organization and delivery of social welfare that took place in the 1980s and 1990s and which were intended to construct a more consumer-like relationship between the users and providers of welfare services. Before looking at these in more detail, however, it is worth standing back and thinking about what might be involved in this consumer relationship. In particular, we need to consider what conditions need to be established to create the possibility of acting as a consumer in relation to welfare services.

ACTIVITY 1.3

Try to define who are the consumers of the following services. Make a note of any problems you have in arriving at such definitions.

Service	Consumers
Health care	
Refuse collection	
Schooling	
Social services	
Police	
Prisons	
Universities	
Income maintenance benefits	

COMMENT

I have always found this a difficult exercise. In some cases I think I can find 'the consumer'. For example, I can imagine myself as the consumer of health care when I visit my GP or go to a hospital. But there are lots of bits of health care (such as public health work) where none of us are 'direct' consumers but we all benefit. The same is true of refuse collection. In the case of other services, it is more difficult to see consumers. For example, are those who are sent to prison the consumers of the prison service? Or should it be those in whose name they have been sent to prison? Finally, even schooling causes me problems. If I think of anyone as a consumer of schooling, it is the child or young person in school. But education policy since the 1980s has been developed on the assumption that parents are the consumers. Why do you think this exercise is so difficult?

■ ■ ■

Schools, hospitals, prisons: who are the consumers?

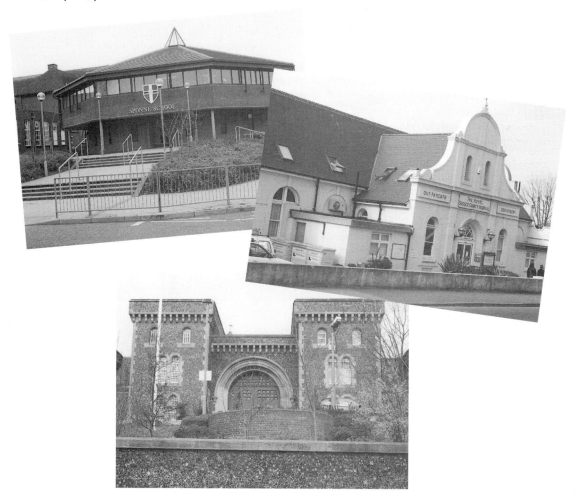

If defining who the consumer is presents some problems, there are other difficulties associated with creating consumerist relationships in social welfare. The image of the 'sovereign consumers' exercising free choice is a difficult one to install in public services. Read Extract 1.3, in which Jennifer Potter has identified some of the central issues and the conditions needed to create consumerism in the public sector.

Extract 1.3 Potter: 'Consumerism and the public sector: how well does the coat fit?'

Consumer theorists argue that there is an imbalance of power between those who provide goods and services, and those for whom they are provided. The former possess all the advantages of corporate power and organization, resources, and political influence. The latter, in the market-place at least, have the choice of buying or not buying a product or service, and – where competitive markets exist – of choosing according to their own preferences. They carry weight, therefore, only as the sum of their individual choices.

To shift the balance of power in favour of consumers, those representing their interests have isolated five key factors which provide a structural underpinning of consumerism. These are the principles of access, choice, information, redress and representation. People must first of all have access to the benefits offered by a product or service (without access, they cannot 'get in'). Their choice of products and services must be as wide as possible to establish some measure of consumer sovereignty, and they need as much information as possible, both to enable them to make sensible choices, and to make the fullest possible use of whatever it is they are seeking. They will also need some means of communicating their grievances when things go wrong, and receiving adequate redress. Finally, they need some means of making sure that their interests are adequately represented to those who take decisions affecting their welfare.

These five tenets were first developed in relation to goods and services sold in the market-place. Consumer choice plays a key role here. People have different requirements and preferences, differing ability to pay, and different views on what constitutes value for money. Where choice exists, individuals can influence the profits and (one assumes) the behaviour of producers by selecting goods and services with the right mix – for them – of price and quality. The existence of competition tends to work in favour of consumers by operating to keep prices down and quality up for each mix that is produced.

[...] Most public services are provided because they are considered to be in the public interest, and working for the public good. They are broadly of two kinds: those designed to give people access to services they would not otherwise be able to enjoy, and those concerned with some form of social control. At the same time, the resources of the public sector are finite and limited, and distributed as an act of political will. This creates an immediate dilemma for the pure application of consumer principles. On the one hand, the nature of public services suggests they are of the utmost importance to those consumers who want to use them; on the other hand, the interests of individual consumers must constantly be juggled against the interests of the community as a whole, and of the other groups who make up that community. Although Stewart and Clarke (Local Government Training Board, 1987) are right to stress, in their development of the public service orientation for local government, that the primary purpose of public services has to be service for the public, deciding what is meant by the 'public' in each particular case presents an immediate problem.

Reference
Local Government Training Board (1987) *Getting Closer to the Public*, Luton, LGTB.

(Potter, 1988, pp.149–51)

Potter identifies five central conditions associated with consumerist initiatives in relation to public services: access, choice, information, redress and representation. Most of these are widely shared by writers dealing with consumerism (although the last is more ambiguous, since it appears to blur the 'exit' versus 'voice' distinction discussed earlier). However, I was surprised to see something missing that struck me as being essential to becoming a consumer. This was the matter of 'resources' or 'capacity' or, to put it more crudely, money. Earlier in the chapter I mentioned the idea of the 'cash nexus' in relation to the process of exchange and consumption. The consumer role seems to centre on the exchange of money for goods or services. Why do you think it is not mentioned here?

COMMENT

The question of money has always been a problematic issue for those arguing for a consumerist version of social welfare provision. For some, the issue is quite straightforward. Reducing taxes allows people to decide how to spend their own money. They can then go out and buy whatever medical, educational or insurance provisions they want. If they fail to buy what they need, that is their problem and the 'nanny state' should not try to rescue them from the consequences of their own choices. This view leaves only a residual question about what to do about those who are too poor to exercise choice in the market-place. Some people simply cannot afford to be consumers. The classical answer to this problem is that of the Poor Law: the benefits or services provided by public authorities or the state should be of a level and quality sufficiently low to dissuade all those but the absolutely desperate from relying on them. In summary terms, this fundamentalist approach to minimal state provision and maximum individual spending choice treats welfare as a matter of individual needs and wants. It sometimes treats individuals as part of families, for whose well-being the head of the household makes choices. There are no 'social' considerations, either in terms of the collective benefits of all being educated or free from contagious disease, or in terms of the inequalities in the amount of money available to be spent on 'welfare'.

choice

■ ■ ■

To move beyond this rather basic economic individualism opens up other sorts of problems, precisely of a 'social' kind. What forms of welfare provision must people be compelled to contribute to and consume? Should everyone contribute to the costs of educating young people? Should all young people be forced to receive education? Should everyone contribute to the costs of controlling illness? Should people who are ill be forced to consume health services? These issues concern matters of collective compulsion. Other social dimensions concern whether or not economic inequalities should be reproduced or redressed by welfare systems. Should having more money enable you to buy more health-care services, more education, a bigger pension? As a consequence, there are arguments over whether markets in welfare services should be 'open markets' (in which people can spend what they wish to achieve a level of provision they want) or 'closed markets' (in which the state provides a voucher that individuals can choose how to spend). There are, of course, possible variations around these two polar types – for example, being able to 'top up' vouchers with one's own income or having 'positively discriminating' vouchers, so that poor people receive larger vouchers to compensate for a lack of money or other social inequalities. These issues begin to hint at why the issue of money is a recurrent difficulty for initiatives aimed at creating consumerism in social welfare.

To some extent these are general social policy questions about the purposes, costs and outcomes of welfare provision. But the figure of the 'consumer' poses them in very sharp and distinctive ways. We understand consumerism in relation to private consumption: we 'know' that money allows us to exercise choice. We also know (or at least suspect) that more money tends to provide more choice. In the context of social welfare, consumerism, choice and money form an uneasy mixture. Perhaps as a result, the developments towards consumerism in social welfare have tended to be partial, limited and often stronger on the rhetoric of choice than its practice.

Consumerism stresses choice as the primary value. In the context of social welfare, what other values or objectives might challenge the value of promoting choice?

Despite these problems, the late 1980s and 1990s saw a range of welfare reforms that claimed to promote a more consumerist orientation in welfare services in the UK. The earliest of these was the 'right to buy' scheme for tenants of local authority housing, which addressed the issue of ownership versus renting for such tenants (as referred to in the extract from Williamson; see also **Pryke, 1998**). Subsequent reforms in schooling, higher education, health services and social care were announced as creating the conditions of choice under which people could act as consumers of social welfare.

What is clear is that there are tensions about how to evaluate or interpret even the limited versions of consumerism that have been introduced into social welfare. For some, the 'customer relations' aspect of consumerism is seen as hiding unchanging or even worsening benefits and services. It may help to cool expectations, disappointment or even anger on the part of service recipients. For others, even these 'weak' versions of consumerism have put pressure on welfare-providing organizations to take their users' needs and views more seriously. In the context of organizations which generally considered 'they knew best' and treated users in imperious or paternalistic ways, even small shifts towards consumerism may be welcome (Hambleton and Hoggett, 1993; Clarke and Newman, 1997, Chapter 6).

Both these positions also influence views on whether the changes have been 'harmful'. To those critical of bureaucratic and professional paternalism, even limited consumerism has meant a step in the right direction and has opened up possibilities of going further. Critics, however, have tended to stress the way in which little power has moved to the recipients of services or benefits. Some have also argued that using the language of consumerism conceals a fundamental difference between commercial markets and public services. In commercial settings,

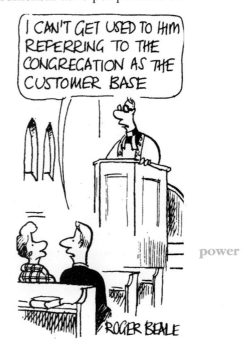

power

increasing demand for your product or service is usually a desirable position, enabling increased profitability. For most public services, rising demand is a problem, because demand is a cost rather than a source of income, and the capacity of the service is limited. Thus, growing health needs constitute a problem for the NHS (rather than an entrepreneurial opportunity). Within limited resources, services come to be rationed and 'demand' has to be managed downwards. Harrow and Shaw point to the possibilities of getting rid of, rather than attracting, consumers:

> A further major factor for public services impinging upon consumer-oriented responses is the extent to which, unlike many companies vying for consumer loyalty, customers of one service will also be customers of another; and that, especially for stretched services, far from seeking to *retain* customers, they may wish – and plan – to pass them on.
>
> (Harrow and Shaw, 1992, p.120)

There is a further tension about consumerism that touches on the relationships between the public and welfare organizations. Do members of the public identify themselves as, or want to be treated as, consumers (or customers)? Does it vary between types of service?

4.1   Chartering a new course?

Many of these ideas about the consumer or customer model of welfare services and the reform of public sector organizations were condensed in the outbreak of 'charters' during the 1990s. The Conservative government introduced the

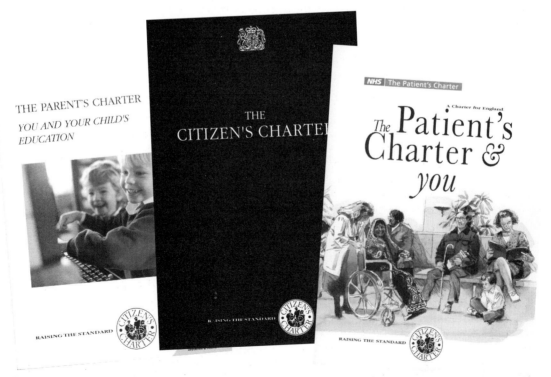

The 1990s saw a proliferation of charters

Citizen's Charter in 1991, drawing on a model of service charters that had emerged in local government. The Charter was then reproduced in a variety of service-specific charters: the Patient's Charter in health services, the Parent's Charter in education, and so on. Some of the significant issues about the 'consumerist' cast of such charters are summarized in Extract 1.4 by Christopher Pollitt.

Extract 1.4 Pollitt: 'The Citizen's Charter: a preliminary analysis'

The White Paper *The Citizen's Charter: Raising the Standard* was published in July 1991. It was particularly closely associated with the then new Prime Minister, John Major. His introduction stated that: 'I want the Citizen's Charter to be one of the central themes of public life in the 1990s'. Eighteen months later, in the *First Report* on the Charter, Major reaffirmed that he envisaged the Charter as a 'ten year programme of radical reform' (Prime Minister, 1992).

There have been a number of (slightly varying) attempts to summarize what the Charter is all about. In *the Citizen's Charter: First Report: 1992* a list of six 'principles of public service' is offered:

- Setting, monitoring and publication of explicit *standards*.
- *Information* for and openness to the service user.
- *Choice* where practicable, plus regular and systematic *consultation* with users.
- *Courtesy* and helpfulness.
- Well publicized and easy-to-use *complaints procedures*.
- *Value for money*.

Each public service or agency has been asked to develop its own charter(s). At the time of writing, there were more than 30 of these, covering most of the public services and some public utilities. Among the most publicized were the *Parent's Charter* (schools), the *Patient's Charter* (hospitals) and the *British Rail Passenger's Charter* ...

As with any new programme, it is instructive to ask who has been given responsibility for what. This may yield a first indication of whose power and authority has been enhanced and which groups have been marginalized or left out. The official version of what is happening is quite clear – management is being decentralized and users are being empowered. Hence: 'The Citizen's Charter is about giving more power to the citizen' (Prime Minister, 1991, p.2). 'Above all the Charter is giving the citizen a real voice' (Prime Minister, 1992, Foreword). 'Front line managers must be made responsible for quality ... Central prescriptions, whose prime focus is to ensure fairness and legitimacy, must be confined to broad principles, and must go alongside maximum flexibility at local level ...' (Goldsworthy, 1992, p.14 – Goldsworthy is Deputy Director of the Citizen's Charter Unit).

In practice, of course, matters are not so simple. The Charter was itself a central initiative, is closely associated with the Prime Minister, and is driven and co-ordinated by a central unit. On occasions central prescriptions have already cut across and distorted the priorities of local management – as when the centre decreed that no-one should wait on an NHS waiting list for more than two years. This resulted in huge pressures on local managements to eliminate such long waits by April 1992, an objective which was almost achieved, but only at the cost of increasing the numbers facing waits of less than a year ... Elsewhere there are examples of silent resistance to what were perceived as central impositions. The provisions of the *Parent's Charter* were regarded as irrelevant or worse by some local education authorities and some headteachers, [who] instead of distributing the leaflets to parents as asked, quietly left them in their boxes in the storeroom.

In other cases still, a good deal has been shaped by local agencies (though that is by no means always the same as 'front line management'). Health authorities were required to set local Charter standards, and at the time of writing most have issued mini-charters of their own ... British Rail have devised quite complicated methods for differentiating between railway routes, with those that fail to reach their set standards not being allowed to raise fares by as much as those which have succeeded. Overall, therefore, the Charter exhibits a complex mixture of centralization and decentralization.

However, central/local is only one dimension of organizational power. At each level there are also various groups of actors (politicians, managers, professionals, users, etc.). There is some evidence to support the government's claims that the users' 'voice' is being enhanced, but to propose that as the *dominant* characteristic of 'charterism' would be a singular exaggeration. It is true that 'voice' should be strengthened by the improvement of complaints procedures and by the injection of a lay element into the inspectorates of prisons, schools, social services and the probation service. Yet it would be easy to exaggerate the emphasis on the user's voice. The charter bears many marks of its origins as a manifesto item for a 'new right' Conservative government. One such is the constant emphasis on 'choice' (i.e. the power of exit rather than voice) and on the virtues of privatization and market testing (Prime Minister, 1992, pp.56–66). Taking the charters as a set there is a marked reluctance to countenance any extension to the *collective* voice of service users. This hostility to 'representationalism', especially as manifested in the form of pressure group activity, was well illustrated by an incident in January 1993. The Secretary of State for Education, John Patten, described spokespersons for the Parents Association as 'Neandertalers' and unrepresentative because they criticized some aspects of his educational reforms. The theoretical citizen cherished by the Conservative government is not a member of any pressure group but rather a heroic lone consumer with time, money and information to back up his or her individual choices. This paragon sounds suspiciously middle class – and relatively rare.

But even if we add choice to voice we are still well short of an adequate characterization of the Charter's implications for power relationships. For, like so many other recent developments forced through in the name of the consumer, the Charter is in many ways a charter for managers as much as for users. The standards which are crucial to the entire enterprise are to be set by managers, who are advised to *consult* consumers but are in no way obliged to comply with their wishes ...

Within public service organizations such as hospitals, universities or local authority departments this responsibility to set standards can and does place an extra lever of influence in the hands of senior management as they deal with semi-autonomous professionals and less senior colleagues.

References

Goldsworthy, D. (1992) 'Efficient and effective management in the new Europe', text of speech presented at management seminar, Dublin.

Prime Minister (1991) *The Citizen's Charter: Raising the Standard*, Cm 1599, London, HMSO.

Prime Minister (1992) *The Citizen's Charter: First Report, 1992*, Cm 2101, London, HMSO.

(Pollitt, 1994, pp.9–11)

Now read Extract 1.5, which is taken from the Open University's Student Charter. What sort of relationship between service provider and user is implied in the extract?

Extract 1.5 The Open University: 'Student Charter'

The UK Government's Charter for Higher Education sets out the standards of service and information that students, employers and the general public can expect from universities, and it indicates what can be done if things go wrong.

The Open University has drawn up its own student charter. This charter summarises the standards and framework for your expectations and responsibilities as a student on an Open University taught course. (The needs of research students are addressed by the Code of Practice for Supervisors and Research Students, which is supplied by the Higher Degrees Office.) Although the Open University Student Charter provides a set of benchmarks, it is not a contractual document between students and the University.

The University will review the Student Charter within two years of publication, and any new developments will be incorporated.

The University's commitment to standards

The Open University's commitment to quality in teaching, assessment and student support, as well as to excellence in research, is firmly established. The University offers an extensive, open-learning curriculum, delivered through mixed media and designed to meet the academic and vocational needs of students. The University is working towards the national Investors in People Standard for the training and development of staff, so as to ensure quality and innovation in everything it does.

The University is committed to equal opportunities for all. It is open to every section of the community regardless of background or circumstance, and it is committed to creating conditions whereby all students can participate fully and equally in the University's activities.

The University is a large and complex organisation in which many departments and staff contribute to a variety of services. Within the framework of the Student Charter, each department operates specific standards directly related to the services it provides.

All departments are committed to respond promptly to queries and to reply to correspondence within ten University working days of its receipt. On a more complex issue where a full reply will take longer than this, you will receive an interim reply giving you a contact name and the anticipated timescale for action. On all matters, University staff will act towards you with courtesy and timeliness, and with respect for confidentially. Your academic record with the University will not be discussed with any third party without your written permission.

What you can expect from the Open University
Access, admissions and finance
The Open University plays a leading role in the provision of open, barrier-free access to higher education, and it is committed to broadening such access for people irrespective of their educational background.

If you are enquiring about studying with The Open University, you can expect the University:

- to give you clear and accurate information about Open University courses, costs and the qualifications offered, so as to enable you to make informed choices
- to offer you individual guidance about choosing Open University courses (contact the Student Support and Advisory Service at your Regional Centre)
- to tell you if and how you can obtain credit for any higher education qualifications you may already have (contact the Credit Transfer and Accumulation Office)
- to give you clear instructions about how to pay fees
- to offer you clear and up-to-date information about the availability of Open University financial assistance awards and how to apply for them (contact the Student Support and Advisory Service at your Regional Centre)
- to process confidentially any application for a financial assistance award that you may make and to tell you how to re-apply for future years if appropriate
- to tell you, if you register to study outside the UK, about specific requirements, limitations, costs, and any Open University facilities that may be relevant to your study

The learning environment and academic support

The Open University serves a large and varied student body in diverse locations by means of a range of supported distance-teaching methods.

As a student on a taught course, you can expect The Open University:

- to provide you with teaching materials developed for distance education
- to dispatch these materials to you in time for you to study them according to the course calendar, provided you enrol by the closing date for registration
- to give you information about the study arrangements for your course, including details of study centres and the provision of tuition
- to offer you educational counselling to assist you in choosing a course and to aid your subsequent progress (contact your counsellor or your Regional Centre)
- to provide tutors who will offer you academic support for your studies, for example by marking tutor-marked assignments (TMAs), giving you constructive written comment and letting you know when they are available for contact
- to assess your work fairly and objectively, with internal monitoring for TMAs and external moderation for examinations (see your Student Handbook for details)
- to return your TMAs within four weeks of the submission cut-off date under normal circumstances (if your TMA is not returned within this period, please contact your tutor in the first instance)
- to provide clear and accurate information about the academic regulations and disciplinary procedures, including appeals (see your Student Handbook for details)
- to give you, if you notify your Regional Centre of a disability or specific disadvantage, information and assistance to facilitate study with the University
- to publish and implement the University's policy on equal opportunities, and its code of practice on harassment
- to operate a safety policy that ensures, so far as is reasonably practicable, the health and safety of staff and students while on University activities
- to supply (on your written authorisation to your Regional Centre) a confidential reference or information about your studies with the University

- to provide (on your written authorisation to your Regional Centre) prompt responses to legitimate queries from your sponsor or employer if you are conducting work-based projects, placements or research, and to identify whom to contact if more information is required.

Representation, participation and quality assurance

The University has established an international reputation for the quality of its teaching and research. It regards the maintenance of quality as of the highest importance, and it therefore strives for continuous improvement in its performance. It is committed to listening to the views of its students, and it particularly values their opinions about courses and tuition. The participation of students is facilitated by the Open University Students' Association (OUSA), which represents student interests on the Senate of the University and on major committees.

You can expect The Open University:

- to give you opportunities (including student feedback questionnaires, committee representation, and a formal complaints procedure) to register your views about your courses, the tuition and the support services
- to tell you about OUSA and its associated societies (see your Student Handbook in the first instance)
- to offer you help, through OUSA, in understanding and exercising your student rights
- to provide you, through membership of OUSA, with the opportunity to participate in making decisions about academic matters and institutional policy.

What The Open University expects from you

The Open University is an educational community which functions on the basis of mutual respect and responsibilities. The UK Government's Charter for Higher Education makes clear that students themselves have certain responsibilities.

To help you get the most out of your studies, the University expects you:

- to observe the University's regulations
- to consult your Student Handbook, which will answer most questions about Open University policies and procedures
- to inform the University of your current address, and to read and respond to communications sent to you by the University or your tutor
- to meet University deadlines (including paying fees according to the published schedules)
- to study the learning materials and make use of the tutoring and counselling support provided
- to help your tutor by submitting assignments on time and by respecting any guidelines about contacting her/him
- to attend residential schools and examinations, if appropriate for your course
- to make known to your Regional Centre, if you wish, any disability or specific disadvantage that may affect your studies and for which the University may be able to make special provision
- to uphold the University's policy on equal opportunities, and its code of practice on harassment
- to act, while on University activities, with reasonable care for your own safety and that of others
- to seek early help and guidance from your tutor, counsellor or Regional Centre if things seem to be going wrong.

What to do if these standards are not met

If you feel that any of these standards has not been met, you should in the first instance contact the most obvious source of the service (for example, your tutor if your TMA is returned late, or the office concerned if you have not received a reply to a query). If you are not sure whom to contact, you should consult the section 'Sources of information and advice' in your Student Handbook to find out where to address your concern, or you can ask your Regional Centre. The telephone number/address of your Regional Centre is in your Student Handbook. Usually the situation can be put right immediately. However, if you are dissatisfied with the response you receive, you may wish to register a formal complaint.

Complaints

Just as your comments, either positive or negative, are valued by the University, complaints are also considered to be an important source of information which helps to maintain standards and make improvements. The University is implementing a formal complaints procedure and is committed to dealing with complaints thoroughly, fairly and as quickly as possible. If you register a formal complaint, you will be sent within ten University working days of its receipt either a full reply or an interim reply giving you a contract name and a date by which you can expect to hear further.

(The Open University, 1995)

COMMENT

The OU's Student Charter defines a particular sort of service relationship and does so in procedural, rather than content-related, terms. The promises made are, in the main, easy to define and easy to measure. They avoid engaging with the complex problems of 'quality'. The Charter is also interesting for the way in which it specifies how a 'responsible' consumer of the service is expected to behave.

■ ■ ■

Charters have been one of the central means of defining the relationships that prevail between the service providers and the users or consumers of those services. They have been remarkable for the ways in which they have avoided specifying rights to services rather than what might be called 'procedural' rights: that you will be dealt with fairly, reasonably and promptly, and that you have the right to complain. These are not 'social rights' – the right to be housed, the right to receive benefits, the right to receive medical treatment, etc. Such social rights might properly have been termed a citizen's charter, but the inflection that is given to citizenship in the official charter is one that reduces it to a consumer model, and a weak version of consumerism at that.

rights

4.2 Consuming welfare

The weakness of welfare consumerism can be seen if we look in more detail at some of the processes involved in specific services. The introduction of markets in health and social care were intended to create competition, choice and a more central role for the individual consumer of such services. In practice, the competition is in relation to purchasers of services who are themselves public sector organizations rather than direct users of the services. Thus, in the market-creating reforms of the health service, the 'purchasing function' was performed on behalf of users by a combination of health authorities and fund-holding general practitioners (GPs) who contracted with service-providing organizations for health provision. This may have made the services more responsive to the needs or wishes of individual patients, but there was nothing in the process to guarantee this. Here, as in other service innovations, the direct user was represented by a 'proxy customer' – the health authority or GP who commissioned or contracted for services (Clarke and Newman, 1997, pp.114–15; **Langan, 1998**).

A similar pattern was visible in the organization of community care, with the user's needs being assessed by a care manager who assembled or purchased an 'appropriate' package of care (Langan and Clarke, 1994; **Barnes, 1998; Pinkney, 1998**). The legislation gave individuals the right to be assessed; it did not guarantee rights to services. As with the charter initiatives discussed above, there were procedural rights and rights to complain. Consumer choice, in the form of parental choice, also featured extensively in the education reforms of the 1980s and 1990s (**Fergusson, 1998**). Studies of how such 'consumers' went about exercising choice demonstrate that consumers are socially constructed in a number of ways**.**

ACTIVITY 1.6

You should now read Extract 1.6, which is from a study of parental choice in education published in 1995. It examines the ways in which (a) 'consumers' are socially positioned and differentiated before they make their choices, and (b) the choices that are available are implicated in the production and reproduction of social differences and inequalities.

Extract 1.6 Gewirtz et al.: 'Choice and class – parents in the market-place'

At the level of political rhetoric, parental choice of school is presented as a mechanism which will extend personal freedom whilst making schools more responsive to their 'consumers'. Embedded within this rhetoric are caricatured versions both of how parents choose and of the effects of those choices … [M]ost parental-choice research and commentary may be divided into two types. The first type treats choice as a decontexualized, undifferentiated and neutral mechanism. This research is itself caught up within the discourse of market theory; the meanings and processes of choice and the constraints upon it for different families are glossed over. The only interest in difference appears to be that of difference in the criteria used or in the 'availability' of choice. The second body of research and writing on parental choice takes matters of difference more seriously, indicating that choice systems discriminate against working-class families … We begin, though, by briefly describing how the concept of 'choice' is being constructed in the public arena both by its advocates and by a growing body of popular texts aimed at helping parents choose schools.

Conservative advocates typically set parental choice within the wider ideology of the market and wider discourses of choice. They present it as fairer than planned provision, because it is 'classless': everyone has the opportunity to choose and to decide upon the 'best' providers of goods and services to meet their needs (but planned interventions continue nonetheless). Greater choice is in itself 'a good thing' because it extends individual freedom. However, such freedom requires individual endeavour, it has to be 'earned', and central to market choice is the assumption that responsible parents will invest a great deal of energy in ensuring that they have made the right choice. Opportunity and responsibility are the keywords here. In *The Parent's Charter* (DES, 1991) choice is powerfully promoted as a personal matter, a question of individual parents taking responsibility for their children's educational future: 'You have a duty to ensure that your child gets an education – and you can choose the school that you would like your child to go to. Your choice is wider as a result of recent changes' (1991, p.8). These new rights, duties and responsibilities are all welded together into a 'language of choice' which has a very overt political role. Parents, or at least a significant number of parents, will need to exercise their individual choices. They will need to actively choose a school rather than allow 'allocation by default'. This appeal to parents to 'consume' education idealizes 'responsible consumerism', both typified and encouraged by the steady growth in consumer magazines and consumer programmes on TV and on the radio, all promoting the merits of being a responsible, rational consumer. In this respect *The Parent's Charter* is both *of* and *in* the social and political context, it emerges from and feeds the ideology of the market and discourses of choice, as well as actively encouraging choice as a right and seeking to construct an image of the responsible parent as one who will display the characteristics of the ideal consumer. This promotion of educational consumerism has spawned the publication of the *Good State Schools Guide* (Clarke and Round, 1991), the schooling-as-product equivalent of the 'consumer's bible', *Which?* Serialized in *The Observer* colour supplement and widely reported in the press, the book aims to identify 300 schools 'which are testimony to the *best* in state education' (emphasis in the original). It includes a seven-page guide, 'What parents need to know', which details parental rights (to choice), types of school, getting local information from the LEA and the school (prospectuses, exam results, visits – what to ask and what to look at), all intended to 'assist you in mounting the ladders and avoiding the snakes' (Clarke and Round, 1991, p.13). This call to consumerism is equally evident in the publicity accorded to 'league tables' and the appearance, in 1992, of other newspaper 'guides' to schools (*The Sunday Times* magazine; *The Independent*; *The Evening Standard* magazine) – now annual publications.

Opponents of educational markets have pointed out that the rhetoric of Conservative advocates of the market obscures the way in which choice systems privilege certain sorts of families and disadvantage others. A wealth of critical commentary accompanied the Education Act 1988, predicting the emergence of a tiered education system, in which working-class children in the cities would get the worst deal ... Furthermore, there has been a growing of body of research on parental choice both in the UK and the USA which supports the contention that educational markets are class-biased. First, the evidence suggests that where oversubscribed schools are allowed to select pupils, modes of selection tend to favour children from middle-class backgrounds. Second, where choice systems operate, research shows that middle-class parents do more choosing than working-class ones. Edwards *et al.* (1989, p.172) found in their study of the Assisted Places Scheme that whilst 'the scheme has certainly benefited large numbers of low income families', children of professional and middle-class parents were predominant amongst place holders. More than half of their sample of 90 parents of assisted place pupils had themselves attended selective or independent secondary schools (1989, p.171). They conclude that 'in the first year of the policy, parental choice was inequitable, in that take-up was more common among better educated parents and those of higher social class' (1989, p.213) ...

Our contextual analysis of choice and class goes to the heart of the ideology of the market and the claims of classlessness and neutrality. Choice emerges as a major new factor in maintaining and indeed reinforcing social-class divisions and inequalities. The point is not that choice and the market have moved us away from what was a smoothly functioning egalitarian system of schooling to one that is unfair. That is crude and unrealistic. There were significant processes of differentiation and choice prior to 1988 (within and between schools). Some skilful and resourceful parents were always able to 'work the system' or buy a private education or gain other forms of advantage for their children. But post-1988, the stratagems of competitive advantage are now ideologically endorsed and practically facilitated by open enrolment, the deregulation of recruitment and parental choice. Well-resourced choosers now have free rein to guarantee and reproduce, as best they can, their existing cultural, social and economic advantages in the new complex and blurred hierarchy of schools. Class selection is revalorized by the market ...

Conclusion

We began ... by indicating the complexity of parental choice of school but we can end it by pointing to at least two very simple and straightforward conclusions. First, choice is very directly and powerfully related to social-class differences. Second, choice emerges as a major new factor in maintaining and indeed reinforcing social-class divisions and inequalities. Again, in stating that, we do not seek to celebrate or romanticize the *past* here. There is a degree of significant continuity in the crucial role played by social class in educational opportunity. The point is that one set of class-related processes is replaced by another set. The 'balance sheet of the class struggle' over educational goods is changed. Choosing is a multifaceted process and there are clear indications here of class, 'race' and gender dimensions to choice. That is, despite some commonalties, the meanings (and implications) of choice vary distinctively between classes: 'different classes have different ways of life and views of the nature of social relationships which form a matrix within which consumption takes place' (Featherstone, 1992, p.86). Where most recent analyses of class differentiation in education have stressed the work of selection and allocation done by schools and teachers, here selection and differentiation is produced by the actions of families. The onus is now more on the 'classified and classifying practices' of the proactive consumer. Education is subtly repositioned as a private good. The previous interrupters of class schooling (ineffective as they often were), like comprehensives with balanced intakes and mixed-ability grouping, are now being displaced. The group rules of the class struggle over educational opportunity have been significantly changed.

The use of cultural capital in the decoding of schools and interpretation of information and in the 'matching' of child to school is a crucial component of choosing and then getting a school place, although economic capital is also important, most obviously in relation to the independent sector. Here we can see the actual realization of social advantage through effective activation of cultural resources ... By linking biography to social structure, the analysis of school choice in relation to class and capital also illuminates the reproduction of class position and class divisions and points up the changing form and processes of class struggle in and over the social field of school choice.

References

Clarke, P. and Round, E. (1991) *The Good State School Guide*, London, Ebury Press.

DES (1991) *The Parent's Charter*, London, Department of Education and Science.

Edwards, T., Fitz, J., and Whitty, G. (1989) *The State and Private Education: An Evaluation of the Assisted Places Scheme*, Lewes, Falmer Press.

Featherstone, M. (1992) *Consumer Culture and Postmodernism*, London, Sage.

(Gewirtz *et al.*, 1995, pp.20–3, 55–6)

social
inequalities

This extract is significant for suggesting how forms of consumerism can reproduce
social inequalities even where there is no 'cash nexus'. How school choices are
made and with what consequences reflects unequal distributions of 'cultural capital'
as well as economic resources. Class inequalities include, and can be reproduced
through, inequalities of valued cultural resources (sets of skills, knowledges,
competencies and elements of personal or interpersonal style) that affect educational
selection. In the process, some parents are better placed to make the 'right' choices
and better placed to be seen by schools as the 'right sort' of parent.

■ ■ ■

Some of these issues about how groups may be differently placed in relation to
the act of consumer choice and the identity of being a consumer are taken up in
Extract 1.7. In this extract John Baldock and Clare Ungerson explore how stroke
victims who need social care on discharge from hospital find different ways of
becoming 'consumers'.

ACTIVITY 1.7

You should now read Extract 1.7 by Baldock and Ungerson. As you do so, think
about the different ways of being a consumer that they identify. You might also
think about why some of the people they surveyed found the consumer role strange.

Extract 1.7 Baldock and Ungerson: 'Becoming a consumer of care'

Local social services must provide dependent people with a needs-based
assessment and they must consult with them and their carers about the provision
of care. It is these aspects that have led to debate about participation, consultation
and empowerment. However, the Act does not give a right to care, only a right to
assessment. Cash limits are likely to force local authorities to complement needs-
based rationing with more explicit means-testing. Traditionally the principle
determining the allocation of local personal social services has been one of need
rather than income. Some LAs continue to insist this remains the case for community
care services. Many, however, are being forced to offer no more than advice to
people above fairly minimal income thresholds. An increasing majority of people
will have to seek their care in the private, voluntary and informal sectors.

Yet relatively little attention has been paid to whether the public are likely to find
the new community care system acceptable and usable and to investigating how
far people will have to change their expectations and behaviour in order to benefit
from the new arrangements. Despite the rhetoric of consumerism, not much effort
had gone into discovering the consumer response to the new community care
product.

Moving across the map of care

Amongst the choices or decisions that the people in our sample appeared to find
difficult, at least initially, were: paying independent professionals such as
physiotherapists; buying private home help; asking family, friends and neighbours
for assistance; paying neighbours and friends; paying members of their own
families; joining voluntary groups and taking advantage of voluntary services such
as speech therapy. In a more general sense these people often found it hard to
grasp or to accept that unless they initiated the use of some of these options nothing

else would happen. For some their inaction was explained by a form of resignation or fatalism but for others apathy was not the problem but rather uncertainty or fear that these sorts of consumption decisions would in some sense be unwise, inappropriate or risky.

Amongst the choices made more readily and frequently were: paying for and arranging forms of transport; paying for alterations and extra equipment for their homes (extensions, alterations, stair lifts); paying for help in the garden; and negotiating those parts of free NHS services that they wanted and avoiding those they did not. In these cases our samples were less surprised that they needed to act and make choices, in other words they expected to behave as consumers.

This is inevitably a very crude summary of complex and evolving patterns of care consumption. Where some people had difficulty others seemed to find the same choices easy and obvious, but overall the journeys people made, as consumers, across the map of care were slow, painful and oddly constrained.

It might be observed that most of the difficulties had to do with making payments to others and so a certain reluctance could be thought to be rather inevitable. However, payment itself was rarely the problem. People in this sample were ready to change their spending patterns. The shock of a stroke is deep; the impact on daily household routines is substantial when people return home to find they can no longer do many of the ordinary things (dress, bathe, drive, talk) that they hitherto had done without a thought. In the face of this trauma people were ready to make big adjustments to their spending patterns and to draw on long held savings. In a number of cases they made substantial, and possibly unwise, expenditure decisions almost as a reflex action. Spending money itself was not the problem ...

By the end of period they had, in each case, to some extent established care régimes that fitted with their expectations about what was right and possible, that were consonant with their pre-existing scripts about how life is lived. They had also, in a variety of ways and to varying degrees, learnt and adapted to new ways of living their lives. As we hope we have shown, these were difficult lessons, or scripts, to learn and required, for some more than others, difficult adjustments. They had had to learn to do things that went 'against the grain' rather than with it.

How are we to characterize the varieties of 'script' according to which people reached decisions (or non-decisions) about how they would live with their new disabilities? We are not seeking to explicate their ideological commitments, such as support for freedom or justice, opposition to poverty or racial discrimination, but rather what sociologists have called 'norms' and 'intermediate values' which drive choice in their everyday lives. Here we would suggest the use of a term first used by Alexis de Tocqueville in his early 19th century study of America. He drew attention to what he termed the *mores* ('*moeurs*') of daily life. He characterized these as:

> Habits of the heart; notions, opinions and ideas that shape mental habits; the sum of moral and intellectual dispositions of people in society; not only ideas and opinions but habitual practices with respect to such things as religion, political participation and economic life.

> (Bellah *et al.*, 1988, p.37)

In a recent and very influential study of the culture and character of American life, a group of sociologists has built upon this idea to construct a typology of 'habits of the heart' (Bellah *et al.*, 1988). Here we attempt to use the same approach to capture the variety of behaviour in the care market amongst our sample.

Figure 1, 'Habits of the heart', describes the two axes. The horizontal axis describes the degree to which the stroke survivors and their carers expected their care to be provided from their own resources or from some kind of collective provision; it distinguishes an individualistic from a collectivist view of welfare. The vertical axis measures people's views of how active they would need to be in order to obtain services; it is a measure of participation. Thus, the diagram presents a model that distinguishes four types of disposition towards the provision of care at the beginning of our study: consumerism, welfarism, privatism and clientalism. What we are presenting are 'ideal types' of care consumers. Rarely were any of our sample solely of one category or another. The function of ideal types is to represent the theoretical range of individual examples. No particular individuals or households corresponded exactly to one or another of the categories; in fact most cases demonstrated elements of each. We shall characterize the qualities of each category by constructing cases that typify them but which are no more than composites of cases we found in our sample.

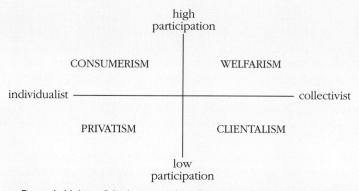

Figure 1 Habits of the heart: modes of participation in the care market

Consumerism

At its extreme this is a view that expects nothing from the state and intends to arrange care by actively buying it in the market or providing it out of household and family resources. There were relatively few examples of this view in our sample. Such people were not ignorant of public provision but were sceptical about whether it would suit them. They might doubt its quality but more often they found it inconvenient and time-consuming to use. For example they objected to the inflexibility of the day-hospital or, at the other extreme, the uncertainty about who would come and when in the case of public domiciliary services. Clearly this is a view which is easier to hold if one has enough money to pay for what one wants but it was not a position limited only to the better off in our sample. People in this category are used to the control and autonomy that being a customer brings and do not like the uncertainty about who is in charge that using voluntary or public services may bring. Thus we found some people with low incomes who would always prefer a private, for-payment arrangement where possible. For example one elderly couple, both of whom were disabled, appeared to have over the years established very reliable relations with a local taxi-driver, a local jobbing builder, a nearby grocer and a butcher (both of whom would deliver) and a number of neighbours who would do odd tasks for payment. For quite small amounts of money this couple appeared to be able to obtain very prompt and flexible attention which they could control. Their 'instincts' were always to use their own initiative. They did not wish to be indebted to anyone and they regarded the increasingly occasional visits of social workers or community nurses as almost purely social events. It must be added that these two people were immensely charming, even jolly; their 'business relationships' had a large non-commercial component.

Privatism

People who fell largely into this category did the least well in terms of support. Many sociologists have commented on the growth of what has been termed 'privatism' in British life (for a summary see Saunders, 1990, pp.275–82). It is associated with owner occupation and thus, in retirement, quite often with moving to a new home in an unknown neighbourhood. Attention is 'devoted overwhelmingly to home and family based life rather than to sociability of a more widely-based kind' (Goldthorpe *et al.*, 1969, p.103). Privatism has also been closely associated with the growth of mass consumerism: 'Ordinary people now demand ever-increasing amounts of consumer goods which they place and use in their own homes. The result is that external and community facilities become marginal to their way of life (Saunders, 1990, p.277). This is a rather passive form of consumerism where most of the work is done by the producers and retailers and requires little initiative from consumers other than the act of purchase itself.

Such a privatized existence may work well when people are fit and the things they want are the products of mass consumerism. When they become ill and dependent and require products and services that are not available 'off the shelf' they have much more difficulty. In our sample these people had tended to refuse help when it was initially offered at the point of discharge. In some cases they very determinedly would not accept an assessment or any care management. They strongly valued their autonomy and would say things like 'we've never depended on other people. We've always looked after ourselves'. At home, as the months went by, we found them increasingly puzzled, embittered and, in some cases, frightened. Few of the skills and attitudes they had accumulated during their fit years seemed to serve them well now. What they needed was not advertised nor available in the ready way of the consumer goods they were used to buying. Neither were they accustomed to the ways of the voluntary and community-based support system. Some found their few unavoidable encounters with neighbours or voluntary help very difficult. For example, one carer-wife whose husband had always done the driving, found the process of negotiating her way round the local parish lift scheme quite excruciating. She felt her privacy invaded, that she was having to beg and to justify her private choices. In seeking to take advantage of a private and market-based approach to home care, policy makers do not seem to have appreciated how impersonal and passive much of more conventional 'participation' in the market is.

Welfarism

This is a set of attitudes and an approach that is associated with such ideas as citizenship and welfare rights. These are people who believe in the welfare state and their right to use it. This implies the active pursuit of one's entitlements. People in this group tend to be educated, articulate and may well have worked in the public sector. The clearest example in our sample was a retired physiotherapist married to an ex-headmaster. She was impressively effective in obtaining the best of what was available in the public and voluntary sector. By the end of the six months she was attending the day-hospital three times weekly but only for so long as was required to receive the physiotherapy she wanted. She had used an NHS domiciliary dentist and an NHS chiropodist who also visited her at home. She attended the stroke club but had refused an offer from a private domiciliary agency because she 'didn't like their money-making approach'. This stroke survivor's most outstanding, but very rare, characteristic was the way she had very explicitly participated in the assessment made by her care-manager. They had reached a clear agreement on what she needed, what she might need in the future and how she would go about contacting the social worker when necessary. However, much as this whole approach was in tune with a citizenship-based conception of welfare, it was equally obvious that if more than a very few people operated in this way the public sector would rapidly be overwhelmed.

Clientalism

This was a common approach amongst our elderly and often low-income sample. It is the 'traditional' way of using the welfare state: passive, accepting, patient and grateful. These people, unlike the privatists, did not refuse or question what was offered. They are accustomed to using what the welfare state offers, adjusting to its rigidities and accepting its omissions. It is a stance that works well where one's needs are high and manifestly so, such as where the stroke survivor was bed- or chair-bound. One does best if one does not get better; indeed more services will tend to appear the longer one is known to the services and less well one does. However, this approach also brings with it the classic and well-known disadvantages of public provision: it is inflexible and time-consuming. Those services one does receive (day-hospital, home care) are rigid in what they can provide and when.

At the same time the public provision leaves gaps. There were things it could not do; for example, put one to bed late. One wheelchair-bound stroke survivor preferred not to go to bed before about 11pm because otherwise her very frail husband would have to help her to the toilet during the night. Although a care assistant came each evening mainly to help the woman to bed, that is not in fact what happened. In other cases the classic inflexibility of public services was not a matter of timing but rather a bureaucratic inability to deal with a quite simple problem: for instance removing a carpet that made it impossible for an elderly woman to use her walking frame or, in another case, providing a much-promised bed-board that might have allowed the client to sleep and so greatly improve the quality of life of an elderly couple who still shared a double bed.

It was most commonly amongst those in our sample who most nearly fitted this category that we found the puzzling denial of having been assessed or even of having a care-manager where we now know one was very much involved. In its most extreme form, the passivity of this stance seems to hide from people even the organizing and planning that is being done for them. They find the ways of the welfare system and its staff unpredictable and do not attempt to understand or change them.

Conclusion

What has been misunderstood is that effective participation by needy people in the mixed economy of care requires that they change values and assumptions that are quite fundamental to how they have lived their daily lives hitherto and that these 'habits of the heart' are embedded in the social relationships in the wider social institutions (the NHS) that have formed the context of people's lives. Policy makers, in designing the new community care, have tended to use frameworks which are largely incapable of grasping these social dimensions. Managerialist analysis is preoccupied [with] structures of incentives and lines of accountability (Griffiths, 1989). Economistic accounts (Audit Commission, 1992) focus on the efficiency of input mixes in obtaining tightly drawn outcomes. In neither case is there much awareness that the users of community care, or consumers as they are more often called these days, may not accept the product in the form that it is intended or even conceive of it in the same terms.

References

Audit Commission (1992) *The Community Care Revolution*, London, HMSO.

Bellah, R. *et al*. (1988) *Habits of the Heart: Middle America Observed*, London, Hutchinson Education.

Goldthorpe, J.H. *et al*. (1969) *The Affluent Worker in the Class Structure*, Cambridge, Cambridge University Press.

Griffiths, R. (1989) *Community Care: Agenda for Action: A Report to the Secretary of State for Social Services*, London, HMSO.

Saunders, P. (1990) *A Nation of Home Owners*, London, Unwin Hyman.

(Baldock and Ungerson, 1996, pp.16–19; 28–33)

COMMENT

Looked at socially, the identity of the consumer is a complex one. It is located in patterns of expectations, assumptions and common-sense knowledges about how the social world works and one's place within it. Baldock and Ungerson usefully show that being a welfare consumer is not simply a matter of doing 'what comes naturally'. Rather, the identity of being a consumer has to be *constructed*. At the same time, this extract reveals other identities – other stocks of knowledge – about people's relation to social welfare on which people draw. As with the issues raised in the education extract, there is a question about the social consequences of the shift to consumerism. If some groups 'know' – or can quickly learn – about how to be a consumer, what inequalities are produced or reproduced in this form of welfare relationship?

■ ■ ■

Finally in this section, it is worth drawing out some of the main points we have considered. The model of consumerism has been influential in shaping the reconstruction of welfare services in the late twentieth century. Nevertheless, it is difficult to see a fully developed consumerism in any of these reforms. Rather they were characterized by weak versions of organizations getting 'close to their customers' or the role of 'proxy customers' in purchasing decisions. At this level it is important to see the consumer role as a social construct, and one whose image might have been more significant than the practices associated with it (Clarke, 1997). We have also seen that the exercise of the consumer role is socially constructed in other senses. People come to the role of the consumer already constituted as 'social subjects' – they occupy differentiated social positions, to which different material and cultural resources are attached. The 'choice making' that such subjects do can serve to reinforce and reproduce their unequal starting-points, but it makes the social character of such inequalities disappear in the 'magic of the market-place'.

5   Possibilities and problems of the consumer model

There has been a range of responses to the development of this consumerist imagery in social welfare. Some have argued that such developments have not gone far enough and represent an impoverished version of the real consumer role, while others have argued that the consumer model is fundamentally misconceived as a relationship on which to base the provision of social welfare. In this third part of the chapter we will examine some of these conflicting views of consumerism in social welfare. The first of these involves the claim that the shifts in the organization of social welfare have fallen short of creating 'real markets' with 'real consumers'.

5.1   More markets, more choice

For many of the advisors, activists and academics who contributed to the arguments about the need to break up state monopolies of welfare provision, the reforms of the 1980s and 1990s represented rather insipid imitations of markets. The tendency towards centralized control, the role of proxy customers, the (over)regulation of both providers and users by government meant that both the dynamism and the consumer sovereignty of 'real markets' were missing. Organizations like the Institute of Economic Affairs attempted to keep up the pressure to free welfare from state provision:

> 'Half-way' houses, like opting-out by suppliers (schools or local authorities) rather than by consumers (individual parents or patients) and privatising laundering or other secondary hospital services or a 'magnet' hospital or school in each region (which in the USA is the preserve of activist whites), will no longer suffice both because they do not prevail over the producer interests which will resist the further advance to consumer sovereignty and because they lag too far behind the social and technical changes exposed by market forces.
>
> (Harris and Seldon, 1987, p.72)

These arguments reflect proposition 1 offered by Keat *et al.* that we encountered in section 3: only the existence of competing providers effectively enables the consumer to *really* choose. Although these arguments had diminished a little in force by the end of the 1990s (in part because of the replacement of the Conservative government in 1997), there remained a strong lobby of 'pro-market' voices insisting that the only effective means of empowering users in relation to social welfare was to turn them into consumers with effective possibilities of choice and 'exit'.

5.2   Creating the citizen-consumer?

A rather different approach to consumerism had emerged in a number of Labour-controlled local authorities, in part reflecting the origins of 'service standards', 'charters' and the 'customer orientation' within local government. This view has focused on what Dowding and Dunleavy (1996) called the 'point-of-service' interactions as a significant feature of the relationship between local residents

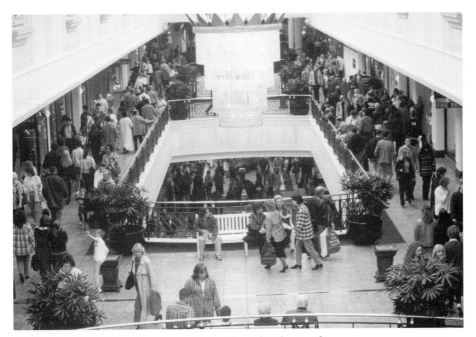

Citizens in a public place, or consumers going about their business?

and the local authority (resembling Keat *et al.*'s proposition 2 about building a consumer-like *relationship*). The contact between what might be described as the local state and the citizen took place in a myriad encounters within schools, libraries, council offices, and so on which could be viewed as 'consumer' encounters. So, rather than rejecting consumerism as tarnished by its association with the Conservative governments of the 1990s, it was argued that local authorities needed to concentrate on the quality of service and interaction issues raised by consumerism as a way of building relationships between consumers/ users/citizens that would strengthen their identification and involvement with the local state.

citizen

ACTIVITY 1.8

You should now read Extract 1.8 by Paul Corrigan. While reading it, think about what problem Corrigan is trying to address in these arguments and why he suggests that relationships of consumption might help to overcome it.

Extract 1.8 Corrigan: 'Recreating the public: a responsibility for local government'

Starting in 1990 a number of local authorities recognised that very specific work needed to be carried out improving the quality of their services. Most of them recognised that this was because we had failed to deliver services which fully reflected people's individual experiences. Most of them recognised that the process of improvement had to directly involve the public.

In Islington, it is clear that if the user of a service did not think they were getting a quality service, then they weren't. It was no longer sufficient, in the world of failed modernism, to claim that a professional could actually assure you that the service you thought was good was in fact bad. The individual consumer was the judge of their own experience. And that individual is not a generic consumer called the public but a specific consumer called an individual. It is they in their idiosyncratic subjectivity that are in charge of the relationship.

In the last few years, councillors have driven much more of the work of public service provision towards the experience of that specific consumer of that specific service. I would suggest that this has had a more profound effect upon the way in which public services have been experienced and provided than all of the analysis of opening up the state to an expanded role of the citizen. There are two major reasons why this is so.

Firstly, as a general part of contemporary social experience, the experience of consumption is ubiquitous. Within the market mechanism most people experience consumption hundreds of times a day. Within many of those experiences – say the supermarket – that consumption experience takes place alongside a great deal of choice – choice within different types of meat for example, and choice within varieties of washing powder. Other consumption experiences may not contain choice – there is only the one train service on the one line, you only have one mortgage once you have it and one gas company to buy from. But even without choice, there are still many experiences of consumption a day. These are very different experiences in different places taking place about different articles but adding up to one of the main experiences every day after every day.

Secondly, in relationship to the local authority, the experience of consumption takes place very much more often than the experience of being a citizen. From the arrival of the rubbish collectors in the morning, through thinking about school for the children, walking down a litter-free street to the aerobic class – walking down that same street in the evening worrying about missing street lights. Day after day relentlessly we consume local authority services.

If they are good we may not notice very much; if that consumption experience is bad, then we notice ferociously … Now it may be the case that people should experience going for a swim as an experience of citizenry, but they don't. It is overwhelmingly experienced as going for a swim …

I am suggesting that within the experience of consumption of a service we have begun to find ways to re-engage with individuals experiencing public services. Because consumption is a frequent everyday experience and allows us to relate strongly to people, we must base our reconstruction on it. It also allows [us] to engage specifically, and through that specificity provides us with the opportunity to overcome the alienation from public services.

Through consumption then we have re-engaged with alienated individuals, for some we have created a real involvement, in that they have been absorbed not only in the experiences of consumption but in the nature of production in the development of that relationship. They are involved in its further development over time. This means that potentially across the country, many thousands of people experience a sliver of empowerment. For many though these are fragmented experiences.

This is good, but I am not suggesting that these fragmented experiences by themselves overcome the alienation of the public from its institutions. They provide the bridge for that transformation but they cannot do it themselves. By themselves, they can recreate the alienation that they are meant to overcome.

For the public, alienation takes a variety of forms. Distance and powerlessness are its main themes. THEY are too far away. THEY tell me what to do. THEY don't care. But the alienation also contains important experiences of fragmentation. Individuals are fragmented from each other, and their experiences are fragmented one from another. For 'a public' to be recreated the experience of individuals needs to be linked not only with state institutions, but with other individuals. The experience of each individual does objectively have similarities that need to be linked to each other.

Therefore it is not enough for local government to collude with the experience that there is no relationship between a swim in the local pool and the rubbish collection. Objectively there is. They are provided from within the same organisation – even if some of the services are being carried out by private contractors, they are provided with public money. Both of them are provided by public money and both are provided by an organisation that has direct citizen relationships. Equally, both of them are provided to your next door neighbour on the same basis as to yourself. They are different services, which generate different experiences, you are different from your neighbour, but they are also part of a wider and a wider experience.

If we want to reconstruct the public then each of these experiences must have the strength to be built upon, each of the differences must have a common thread which can then be woven together. Much of this is in the tactic of the original consumption experience. It is vital, for example, that logos, styles of printing, and methods of communicating have a uniform brand image. Just as large private companies provide a very wide range of goods and services but can have an identifiable relationship constructed through those differences, then the public organisation must do the same.

It is this dialectic between the recognition of great differentiation of the experience of consumption and the consistent experience of the one local government organisation, that is vital. Organisationally, this is how modern organisations are moving. The provision of a wide number of individually distinct experiences of consumption alongside a strong central branding theme of the organisation is the nature of modern organisation.

How will this dialectic evolve for the local authority committed to reconstructing its public? After successfully differentiating the experience of service delivery, if it wants to reconstruct a fragmented public, it must represent itself strongly as a single organisation. The swimming pool provided by a contracted company, the education provided by a locally managed school, the social service by a voluntary organisation and the council tax bills sent by the directly employed officers, are all provided through the powers of a single organisation.

It is vital that the organization of the Authority, alongside the experience of the public, overcomes this appalling fragmentation. At the moment, it rarely does, at the best it has recognised the importance of service differentiation, but it rarely identifies the absolute necessity of re-engaging all of that differentiation and by doing recreating that public.

(Corrigan, 1996, pp.10–14)

COMMENT

Corrigan's argument addresses the alienation or disconnection of people from public services and public organizations. In doing so, he draws on a left-wing critique of traditional public services as paternalistic, controlling and oppressive. Services that treated people as passive recipients who were expected to be grateful for what they got were unlikely to provide a strong base of public support or enthusiasm. He suggests that a public culture could only be rebuilt by focusing on those points of practical intersection between members of the public and the state (the 'points of service') that can provide a basis for people feeling that they have a stake in or an attachment to public services.

■ ■ ■

This is clearly a very different view of the possibilities of consumerism. Rather than seeing it as antithetical to, or even destructive of, a public or collective culture of welfare, Corrigan and others have suggested that by taking people's experience of consuming public services seriously, it might be possible to build on those relationships to renew or recreate a sense of a public realm. This is treating consumerism as the starting-point, rather than the desired end-point, for the reconstruction of public services. In this view, consumerism provides a 'structure of feeling' that has political possibilities for building new collective identities.

5.3   Not just now: the problem of choice

A different challenge to the view of welfare service users as 'consumers' has been developed by a number of analysts who have indicated problems concerning the nature of the consumption process involved. Some of these point to the fact that some services have no direct consumers who can be separated out from the 'general public' (for instance in environmental health provisions); others have collective users rather than, or as well as, individual consumers. Equally, some recipients of welfare services are obliged or forced to receive them, perhaps unwillingly. But even where there are individual consumers who can be clearly identified (such as in health or social care provision) there are some problems about treating this as if it is or should be a site of consumerism. Barnes and Prior (1995) have argued that the point of consumption of many public services is a moment at which people often will not want to act as consumers:

> Public services can be used in conditions which are likely to be experienced as risky, confusing and uncertain. This implies that, at the point of consumption, values such as confidence, security and trust may be more appreciated by users than the opportunity for choice ... A simple notion of choice as selecting between options cannot stand up to systematic analysis of the processes through which people come to receive and make use of welfare services.
>
> (Barnes and Prior, 1995, p.58)

Barnes and Prior argue that the complexity of these processes means that efforts to reform services to make them more responsive to user interests need to address very differentiated types of power and decision-making. These range from how to organize the immediate provision of a benefit or service to a particular user, through planning service design, goals and processes with the collective participation of users, to thinking about how to engage both users and other citizens in the invention, planning and choices associated with social welfare in contemporary society.

5.4 Choices versus rights

The issue of whether 'choice' should be the dominant value in welfare policy has been explicitly addressed by user organizations and disabled people's movements (Croft and Beresford, 1996). Questions about how to shape welfare services raise issues beyond the consumer relationship, even in its fully marketized form. For such groups the central issues concern power, participation and rights or entitlements rather than needs or wants (**Langan, 1998**). At the core of these arguments is the tension between entitlements to being treated as a full and active citizen as opposed to being treated as a diminished person with 'special needs'. Some of these arguments were taken up by Alan Walker in a commentary on the NHS and Community Care Act 1990 (see Extract 1.9).

Extract 1.9 Walker: 'From consumerism to empowerment'

The Griffiths Report, White Paper and National Health Service and Community Care Act all derive from the limited form of supermarket-style consumerism which assumes that, if there is a choice between 'products', service users will automatically have the power of exit from a particular product or market. Of course, even if this is true in markets for consumer goods, in the field of social care many people are mentally disabled, frail and vulnerable; they are not in a position to 'shop around' and have no realistic prospect of exit.

Underlying the consumerist model of social care are two questionable assumptions. It is assumed that monopolies only operate in the public sector. Also it is assumed that the private sector can adequately substitute for the public sector. But, as far as, for example, an older person currently resident in either a public *or* a private home is concerned, her provider *is* the monopoly power because she has no alternative. Having a range of theoretical alternatives will not make the consumer sovereign if she cannot exercise effective choice. Moreover, a financial transition does not necessarily mean the bestowal on the purchaser of either influence or control over the provider. Furthermore, unlike markets for consumer durables, in the field of social care if the private producer goes out of business this will not only have immense human consequences but the public sector will be expected to pick up the pieces. In other words, the private sector exercises equivalent power over users to public providers but it does not necessarily carry the same responsibility.

The only way that frail and vulnerable service users can be assured of influence and power over service provision is if they or their advocates are guaranteed a 'voice' in the organization and management of services. This would, in turn, ensure that services actually reflected their needs. In practice the weak form of consumer consultation pursued under the 1990 Act could consist of no more than an occasional survey among the users together with minimal individual consultation at the point of assessment. (This is certainly the model being offered to local authorities by private management consultants and the signs are that many are adopting it.) Thus despite the rhetoric concerning 'packages of care' and making services more responsive to users, in practice the government's proposals are silent on how user involvement can be ensured and are characterised by old style paternalism.

In contrast to the consumer-oriented model, the user-centred or empowerment approach would aim to involve users in the development, management and operation of services as well as in the assessment of need. The intention would be to provide users and potential users with a range of realisable opportunities to define their own needs and the sorts of services they require to meet them. Both carers and cared-for would be regarded as potential service users. Where necessary the interests of older people with mental disabilities would be represented by independent advocates. Services would be organized to respect users' rights to self-determination, normalization and dignity. They would be distributed as a matter of right rather than discretion, with independent inspection and appeal procedures, and would be subject to democratic oversight and accountability.

What changes in policy are necessary if community care services are to move beyond consultation to empowerment? In the first place it is necessary to recognise that while the private and voluntary sectors may extend choice in social care they cannot substitute for the public sector. Only the public sector can guarantee rights to services. Moreover the motivations of a for-profit private producer are quite different from those of a public sector provider. Although both may provide opportunities to exploit vulnerable people it is only in the public sector that a direct line of enforceable public accountability exists ... It must be said too that, as far as Britain is concerned, the public sector of care is notably more successful at involving users than its private counterpart.

Second, change is necessary in the organisation and operation of formal services. The concept of social support networks is particularly helpful in emphasising the need for formal and informal helpers to cooperate, share tasks and decision making and 'interweave' ... In addition SSDs [social services departments] must develop explicit strategies for the involvement of service users, carers and potential users. The essential ingredients of such a strategy are positive action – to provide users and potential users (or their advocates) with support, skills training, advocacy and resources – so that they can make informed choices, and access – the structures of the agency must afford opportunities for genuine involvement. According to Croft and Beresford (1990, p.14): 'Unless both are present people may either lack the confidence, expectations or abilities to get involved, or be discouraged by the difficulties entailed. Without them, participatory initiatives are likely to *reinforce* rather than overcome existing race class, gender and other inequalities'. Thus user involvement must be built in to the structure and operations of SSDs and not bolted on.

Third, change must be initiated in professional values and attitudes within the formal sector so that cooperation and partnership with service users is regarded as a normal activity. This does *not* mean that service provision must be deprofessionalised if user involvement is to flourish; rather that the role of professionals must change in order to share power with users. This means challenging, to some extent, the traditional basis of professional status and providing for the input of informed user knowledge and preferences, which means finding ways for community members themselves to take part in the development of community care policy – in short, power sharing.

Fourthly, the previous two points suggest a major transformation in training and retraining for social services personnel. Thus the emphasis would shift away from autonomous expertise and individual diagnosis towards skills for working in partnership with service users and their carers, and encouraging community participation.

Finally, user involvement is not a cheap option; it is usually time-consuming and costly. Therefore there is a need for increased resources in the social services not only to improve the choice and quality of services but also to ensure that they provide sufficient space for the direct involvement of users.

Thus if significantly greater reforms were made available it would be possible for some of the reforms contained in the National Health Service and Community Care Act 1990 to be implemented in a progressive way. For example, assessment could be operationalised as an open process designed to explore and create options rather than ration resources. It could be carried out by users themselves or in partnership with social services professionals. Contracts could be used to ensure high standards are maintained, rather than high prices, and that agencies have equal opportunities employment policies and anti-oppressive forms of practice. Quality could be guaranteed by granting users *rights* in terms of both standards and levels of services. But, arguably these sorts of development would alter the main thrust of current community care policy and, therefore, would first require a change of political direction.

Reference
Croft, S. and Beresford, P. (1990) *From Paternalism to Participation*, London, Open Services Project.

(Walker, 1993, pp.221–3)

This view treats consumerism as an ill-fitting image for the purpose, process and practice of welfare services. By focusing only on the 'point of service', consumerism offers an impoverished conception of what welfare is and what rights citizens/users/members of the public might have, or need, in relation to it. Unlike commercial markets, members of the public might also want a say in 'what business' welfare organizations are in, how they go about that business, and how they treat the user at the point of service. *Procedural* rights to being dealt with promptly and fairly may be important, but without other rights guaranteeing benefits, services or forms of treatment, they fail to address the *content* of social welfare.

6   Towards a nation of consumers?

We have moved from arguments that the consumer model ought to define the way forward for the relationship between the public, the state and social welfare to arguments that it cannot sustain an *adequate* conception of that relationship. It is clear that the imagery of the consumer has been extremely influential, both in legitimating the process of welfare restructuring in the 1990s and in reshaping some of the points of contact between members of the public and public services. At the end of the 1990s, the tensions around consumerism remained potent ones for the future of social welfare. It was less clear that consumerism was seen as the single best way – or the only relationship that should be involved in connecting the public, the state and welfare. At the same time, the consumerist shifts of the 1980s and 1990s were, for the most part, firmly established elements of welfare policy and practice, both as consumer choice and consumerist relationships. Perhaps the most striking exception was in the Benefits Agency, where a programme intended to develop a strong 'customer orientation' was abandoned in the mid 1990s in the face of increased government pressure for financial savings.

What is more difficult to assess is whether the figure of the consumer could ever be an adequate basis on which to reinvent the relationship between the people, the state and social welfare. Does this figure create sufficiently strong patterns of relationships and representations to provide a coherent 'structure of feeling' for the future of social welfare?

COMMENT

Here are some of our suggestions about the possible strengths and weaknesses of the figure of the consumer.

Strengths	Weaknesses
It promotes choice	It tends to individualize or privatize
It 'empowers' users	It does not give real rights to welfare
It refers to everyday social roles	Being a welfare consumer is not necessarily what people want
It brings the state and the market closer together	Social welfare is not a simple commodity
It enables individuals and their families to decide on their welfare needs	It enables some people more than others
It envisages a nation of 'freely choosing individuals and families'	It fails to promote solidarity, mutuality or an effective image of 'the people'

The imagery of consumerism has had a very strong appeal that can command attention and attachments among members of the public. It is a potent structure of feeling. In part, this is because consumerism addresses or responds to a range of criticisms of and challenges to the 'old' welfare state. Consumerism addresses New Right concerns about state monopolies over welfare provision and the suppression of competition, choice and individual responsibility. At the same time, consumerism can be seen as responding to challenges from the Left and user groups about the paternalism and concentrations of power in the state (as in Extract 1.8 above). Finally, consumerism can be seen as responsive to issues of social diversity in its claim to be closer to individual needs and wants. In these ways, consumerism appeared as a solution to many of the criticisms of state welfare provision.

Consumerism also commanded considerable support from a number of directions because, Extract 1.2 suggested, it raised issues of *power* and *control*. Consumerism involved an acknowledgement that there were issues of power and control at stake in the provision of welfare, and a recognition that individual recipients of services had genuine concerns, wishes and perceptions of their own needs that were often ignored by welfare providers. It may be that consumerism in practice does not resolve those sorts of problems very effectively, and it may give rise to others. Nevertheless, the appeal of consumerism as an imagery for the relationship between welfare and the public rests on its capacity to take up or engage with these issues of power and control.

At the same time there are other social dimensions of consumerism that account for resistance to it as a form of relationship between the public and welfare. It is worth summarizing these around three main issues: the problem of inequalities; the problem of power; and the problem of society.

Starting with inequalities, consumerism risks producing or reproducing social inequalities. A consumer relationship to welfare provision based on the 'cash nexus' would simply enable those with greater wealth to purchase more, or better, welfare benefits and services. (Of course, this relationship has always existed to the extent that it is possible to purchase benefits and services 'privately', as in schooling or health care.) However, as we have seen earlier in the chapter, even where consumer choices do not involve direct purchasing, forms of social differentiation and inequality can be reproduced through such processes. But because they appear in the form of 'individual choices', the reproduction of social divisions may be more difficult to identify.

social differentiation

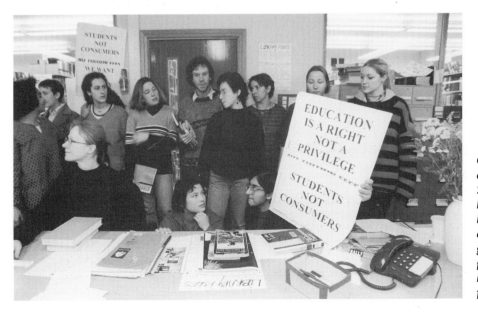

Consumerism: a contested status. Students at the London School of Economics protest against the government's proposal to introduce tuition fees

The question of individual choices is also linked to the *problem of power* in consumerism. Consumerism tends to reduce issues of power and control to matters of individual choice (and even then there may be problems about who gets to make choices). What it neglects, or treats as irrelevant, are wider political processes of power and control – over policy, resourcing and the direction of services and benefits. Consumerism tends to concentrate on 'point of service' matters but, as Walker and others have argued, there are other dimensions of power that are vitally important in social welfare.

Finally, consumerism is a representation of the world as being composed of individual 'choosers', each pursuing their own interests. This is not surprising, given that its theoretical foundations are in neo-classical economics, which deals in individualized agents linked or co-ordinated by markets. Nevertheless, this individualist approach has two significant implications for social welfare. First, in relation to social differentiation consumerism treats diversity as a matter of diversity of individual 'wants'. Second, there is no conception of difference as involving socially structured inequalities (Williams, 1996).

As a result, consumerism makes it harder to address the *problem of society.* Dealing in ideas of individualized and privatized choosing means it is difficult to identify who the *public* is, what the *public interest* might be, or what *collective choices* need to be made. Of course, for the proponents of free markets, this is precisely the point: attempts to 'invent' such collective or public interest interferes with individual choices and their co-ordination by the market. In this view there is 'no such thing as society', but it is an impoverished view of the social realm which by the late 1990s had provoked a backlash against the narrow individualism of consumerism and markets (Clarke, 1996). Consumerism provided a potent structure of feeling that articulated challenges to the old structures of welfare provision. However, its limited view of the public led to a renewed interest in more social and political forms of imagining the relationship between the people, the state and social welfare. In particular, the figures of the 'community' and the 'citizen' became the focus of renewed discussion.

Further reading

This chapter's analysis of consumerism is closely related to the discussion in Clarke and Newman (1997), particularly Chapters 6 and 7. A more detailed exploration of some of the organizational reforms associated with consumerism can be found in Butcher (1995). Some of the issues about consumerism, power, control and citizenship are examined in Barnes (1997).

References

Baldock, J. and Ungerson, C. (1996) 'Becoming a consumer of care: developing a sociological account of the "new community care"', in Edgell *et al.* (eds) (1996).

Barnes, M. (1997) *Care, Communities and Citizenship*, Harlow, Addison Wesley Longman.

Barnes, M. (1998) 'Whose needs, whose resources? Accessing social care', in Langan (ed.) (1998).

Barnes, M. and Prior, D. (1995) 'Spoilt for choice? How consumerism can disempower public service users', *Public Money and Management*, July–September, pp.53–9.

Barry, N. (1991) 'Understanding the market', in Loney, M. *et al.* (eds) *The State or the Market: Politics and Welfare in Contemporary Britain*, 2nd edn., London, Sage.

Butcher, T. (1995) *Delivering Welfare: The Governance of the Social Services in the 1990s*, Buckingham, Open University Press.

Cahill, M. (1994) *The New Social Policy*, Oxford, Blackwell Publishers.

Clarke, J. (1991) *New Times and Old Enemies: Essays on Cultural Studies and America*, London, Routledge.

Clarke, J. (1996) 'Public nightmares and communitarian dreams: the crisis of the social in social welfare', in Edgell *et al.* (eds) (1996).

Clarke, J. (1997) 'Capturing the customer: consumerism and social welfare', *Self, Agency and Society*, vol.1, no.1, pp.55–73.

Clarke, J. and Newman, J. (1997) *The Managerial State: Power, Politics and Ideology in the Remaking of Social Welfare*, London, Sage.

Corrigan, P. (1996) 'Recreating the public: a responsibility for local government', an inaugural lecture, University of North London.

Croft, S. and Beresford, P. (1997) 'The politics of participation', in Taylor, D. (ed.) *Critical Social Policy: A Reader*, London, Sage.

Dowding, K. and Dunleavy, P. (1996) 'Production, disbursement and consumption: the modes and modalities of goods and services', in Edgell *et al.* (eds) (1996).

du Gay, P. (1996) *Consumption and Identity at Work*, London, Sage.

Edgell, S., Hetherington, K. and Warde, A. (eds) *Consumption Matters*, Oxford, Blackwell/Sociological Review.

Fergusson, R. (1998) 'Choice, selection and the social construction of difference: restructuring schooling', in Hughes and Lewis (eds) (1998).

Gardner, C. and Sheppard, J. (1989) *Consuming Passion: The Rise of Retail Culture*, London, Unwin Hyman.

Gewirtz, S., Ball, S. and Bowe, R. (1995) *Markets, Choice and Equity in Education*, Buckingham, Open University Press.

Hambleton, R. and Hoggett, P. (1993) 'Rethinking consumerism in public services', *Consumer Policy Review*, vol.3, no.2, pp.103–11.

Harris, R. and Seldon, A. (1987) *Welfare Without the State: A Quarter Century of Suppressed Public Choice*, London, Institute of Economic Affairs.

Harrow, J. and Shaw, M. (1992) 'The manager faces the consumer', in Willcocks, L. and Harrow, J. (eds) *Rediscovering Public Services Management*, Maidenhead, McGraw-Hill.

Hirschman, A.O. (1970) *Exit, Voice and Loyalty: Responses to Decline in Firms, Organizations and States*, Cambridge, Mass., Harvard University Press.

Hughes, G. and Lewis, G. (eds) (1998) *Unsettling Welfare: The Reconstruction of Social Policy*, London, Routledge in association with The Open University.

Keat, R. and Abercrombie, N. (eds) (1991) *Enterprise Culture*, London, Routledge.

Keat, R., Whiteley, N. and Abercrombie, N. (eds) (1994) *The Authority of the Consumer*, London, Routledge.

Langan, M. (ed.) (1998) *Welfare: Needs, Rights and Risks*, London, Routledge in association with The Open University.

Langan, M. and Clarke, J. (1994) 'Managing the mixed economy of care', in Clarke, J., Cochrane, A. and McLaughlin, E. (eds) *Managing Social Policy*, London, Sage.

Larner, W. (1997) 'Market governance and the consumer', *Economy and Society*, vol.26, no.3, pp.373–99.

Open University (1995) *Student Charter*, Milton Keynes, The Open University.

Pinkney, S. (1998) 'The reshaping of social work and social care', in Hughes and Lewis (eds) (1998).

Pollitt, C. (1994) 'The Citizen's Charter: a preliminary analysis', *Public Money and Management*, April–June, pp.9–11.

Potter, J. (1988) 'Consumerism and the public sector: how well does the coat fit?', *Public Administration*, vol.66, pp.149–64.

Pryke, M. (1998) 'Thinking social policy into social housing', in Hughes and Lewis (eds) (1998).

Walker, A. (1993) 'Community care policy: from consensus to conflict', in Bornat, J., Pereira, C., Pilgrim, D. and Williams, F. (eds) *Community Care: A Reader*, Basingstoke, Macmillan.

Williams, F. (1996) 'Postmodernism, feminism and the question of difference', in Parton, N. (ed.) *Social Theory, Social Change and Social Work*, London, Routledge.

Williamson, J. (1987) *Consuming Passions: The Dynamics of Popular Culture*, London, Marion Boyars.

CHAPTER 2

Community

by Gordon Hughes and Gerry Mooney

Contents

1   Introduction

From concerns about 'problem communities' in the 1960s through to the community care legislation of the late 1980s and 1990s, the idea of community has been a pervasive feature of social policies in contemporary UK society. Furthermore, community was given renewed meaning and vitality in the mid to late 1990s, and this chapter looks at how the idea of community became central to discussions about how social relations are figured and imagined.

'Community' is such an integral part of everyday language and thinking that reference to it tends to pass with little comment. This chapter seeks to problematize this by discussing some of the ways in which the idea of community has been used to represent relations between the individual, civil society and the state. The chapter is about contested representations of community; the ways in which meanings of 'community' have been socially constructed. It is also about the way in which communities are always *imagined* and *reimagined*, as part of the process by which people attempt to make sense of the world.

The main aims of the chapter are:

- To demonstrate that community is a highly contested notion.

- To consider some of the ways in which community has been constructed as a site of policy intervention.

- To explore the ways in which community is used as a means of expressing feelings and identities.

- To examine the competing moral and political discourses of community.

The chapter is organized in two main parts. Section 2 begins by considering ways in which the idea of community has been used both in academic social science and in wider social commentaries. It then discusses three of the ways in which the idea of community has been understood and imagined: as an area of public policy; as a sense of place; and as feelings of belonging. While these are discussed separately, you should bear in mind that they overlap and frequently conflict with and contradict each other. The goal of section 2 is for you to understand that community is something which is forged and made, not fixed. The section also emphasizes the continuing appeal of community as a highly seductive way of making sense of and representing social experiences.

Section 3 explores the question of what community might mean as an orchestrating principle of social policy. Here the discussion focuses on two very different and opposing discourses on community: that of moral communitarianism and that of radical left pluralism. We look at how these two discourses have deployed the notion of community in their political and moral agendas on the future of social policy as well as in the reconstitution of what the Introduction to this book described as 'the national popular'.

2   The seductions of community

2.1   Why community?

Pause for some reflection and consider what images the idea of community conjures up for you.

The idea of community is regularly invoked either as a critique of social life or as a means by which certain relationships and processes can be legitimated. As Raymond Plant (1978, pp.80–1) commented: 'it is used not only to describe or refer to a range of features in social life but also to put those features into a favourable perspective.'

The term's popularity says much about its ambiguity – the fact that it can be used in descriptions and analyses of social processes and relations without requiring clear definition and explanation. After all, common sense tells us what a community is, doesn't it? Many people experience a powerful nostalgia for an imagined past golden age of community life when friends and family lived close by; when doors were always open; when the street was a place of excitement and communality; when people stuck together in times of adversity. But for many, globalization, urban change, economic restructuring, the break-up of 'family life', migration and/or a growing uncertainty about the world in which we live has disrupted 'traditional' senses of community. As we will discover, the idea of community has both a long and troublesome history and a very strong resonance.

Since the 1980s the idea of community has been a central concept in both academic and populist political discourses and in popular media coverage of a wide range of social issues, especially debates about the future of welfare provision and delivery. It is widely used in social and political analysis, as a tool of policy development and as a critique of what has been widely perceived as a rise in social exclusion and fragmentation, and a corresponding breakdown in social cohesion.

From the late 1970s political theory was dominated by liberal individualism, which postulates an autonomous, assertive, rational individual – the consumer – who must be protected from state power and 'public interference' (see Chapter 1). But such ideas did not go unchallenged (Gray, 1995). The Labour government elected in 1997 under Tony Blair has accorded prominence to 'the social', or 'the public', as well as to the individual. Community in this respect implies a rejuvenated civil society, occupying some mid-way point between the state and the market. Appealing to 'community values' thus allows for a reconfiguration of the public sphere after a prolonged attack by the New Right. Advocates of communitarian ideas, in particular, argue that the community rather than the individual (or the state) should be at the centre of both analysis and the prevailing value system (Frazer and Lacey, 1993, p.1). We return to this in section 3.

Other continuing debates about community include the controversy over the consequences of community care strategies, with feminist thinkers in particular criticizing the gendered assumptions which underpin many uses of 'community'; the arguments that community breakdown is a key contributing factor in patterns of rising crime and delinquency; and claims that some communities are being excluded from 'mainstream' social life in a period of increased social polarization and greater social inequality (Campbell, 1993;

Danziger, 1996; Cole *et al.*, 1997). Such claims appear to echo Aneurin Bevan's fears about social segregation in the UK after the Second World War:

> [Y]ou have colonies of low-income people living in houses provided by local authorities, and you have the high income groups living in their own colonies. This segregation of the different income groups is a wholly evil thing from a civilised point of view ... It is a monstrous infliction upon the essential psychological and biological oneness of the community.
>
> (Bevan, quoted in Lansley, 1979, p.183)

Similar arguments and themes tend to recur in different historical contexts, highlighting the continuing potency of community. The language and imagery of community has never been far from those concerned with a variety of social problems and it acts as a recurring reference point from which certain social behaviours and lifestyles can be questioned and marginalized.

The idea of community, then, tends to rest on an emotional appeal to both an imagined past and to an idyllic future (Worsley, 1987, p.238). We may ask whether all agree that community is an unmitigated good thing, underpinned as it is by the central idea that 'people have something in common' (Hill, 1994, pp.34–5), and whether any 'decline' of community, or community 'spirit', is something to be regretted and prevented. It is widely claimed that modern societies such as the UK are characterized by a loss of community, with social life becoming less cohesive as the twentieth century progressed (Lee and Newby, 1983; Johnson, 1994, p.13). This is regarded as especially true of 'traditional working-class communities', which were thought to be characterized by a set of explicit values, such as honesty, solidarity, communality and interdependency (Bornat, 1993, p.23). Such communities, it is argued, were eroded by deindustrialization, urbanization, urban renewal and slum clearance, immigration, out-migration and/or the rise of selfish individualism. 'Loss of community' is a phrase frequently used, as Lee and Newby (1983, p.52) comment, 'in an oblique but poignant way to express the dissatisfaction which many people experience about the quality of life in the contemporary world.' It is argued, therefore, that the longing for community represents a desire for more security in an ever more alienating, globalized world in which local communities have been threatened and undermined.

Perhaps many of these arguments are all too familiar to you. They may reflect your own views. Ideas of community are, after all, a key part of popular social discourse. But note that thus far we have offered no definition of community. The reason for this is simple: community is a particularly elusive and value-laden concept. Hillery (1955, p.117) identified no less than 94 different definitions of community, the only link between them being that 'all of the definitions deal with people.' The ambiguity of the notion of community is part of its seductiveness.

2.2 Community as a site of state intervention

The salience of the idea of community is apparent from even a cursory glance at public sector job titles or department names and roles: community work, community care, community development, community education, community health, community policing.

Community first began to feature strongly in public policy in the 1960s. In

loss of
community
traditional
working-class
communities

58

part this was due to a growing interest by both social scientists and policy-makers in working-class communities in particular in a period of major social change (see section 2.3.1). During the 1960s a number of academic studies and policy reports drew attention to the persistence of social and economic inequality in post-war UK society, together with deepening poverty. Attention was focused on communities where, it was claimed, 'dysfunctional' or 'problem' families susceptible to poverty were to be found. From this period the language of community became firmly established as a means of legitimating state intervention and regulation and, in the process, community was constructed as a site of intervention.

state intervention

Following the designation of certain areas of the urban UK as dysfunctional – defined primarily in terms of poverty, low levels of educational achievement, family breakdown and, increasingly, 'racial problems' – there was a prolonged assault on a number of 'deviant' communities. Community was thus both constructed and regulated through a series of central and local state projects, from the Community Development Projects in the late 1960s to the Comprehensive Community Programmes and the Community Trusts and Community Programmes in the 1970s and 1980s.

By the late 1980s and 1990s the language of community 'participation' and 'partnership' was a key feature of urban programmes in both the UK and the USA (Barr, 1995; Duffy and Hutchinson, 1997). The City Challenge project in England stressed the role of local communities in implementing strategies, but there was even more emphasis on community involvement in the Scottish Office's urban regeneration strategy. New Life for Urban Scotland, launched in 1988, focused on four disadvantaged housing estates in Scotland's major cities (Scottish Office, 1988). This was embedded in a rhetoric of community involvement, with the 'community' supported by full-time community development workers. That such a strategy was fraught with difficulty (Duffy and Hutchinson, 1997; McArthur, 1995; Scottish Office, 1996) does not detract from the ways in which community has been deployed, primarily as a means of legitimating strategies and, in a period of financial constraints and cut-backs, diverting attention from central and local government funding policies towards 'locally made' decisions and 'choices'.

For Cochrane (1986, p.51), central and local governments (and a plethora of other agencies in the urban regeneration business) have used community 'as if it were an aerosol can, to be sprayed on to any social programme, giving it a more progressive and sympathetic cachet.' The language of community configures the *imagined territory* upon which programmes and policies should act (Rose, 1996, p.331). In turn, the subjects of intervention are also defined and redefined. Community, then, is a key means of representing, problematizing and intervening in a number of policy areas. For Rose:

> Communities become zones to be investigated, mapped, classified, documented, interpreted, their vectors explained to enlightened professionals-to-be in countless college courses and to be taken into account in numberless encounters between professionals and their clients, whose individual conduct is now to be made intelligible in terms of the beliefs and values of 'their community'.
>
> (Rose, 1996, p.332)

The deployment of community through a wide range of social policies is instrumental in both constructing and reproducing community as an imagined figure through which political strategies are channelled and given authenticity.

59

In the process, community as an element of the national popular is strengthened. But while the appeal to community is clear, the practice is more problematic. Who constitute the community to be 'empowered'? What community should provide 'community care'? Who will deliver 'punishment in the community'? Politically, community may be attractive; organizationally it has proved to be highly problematic. In part this is due to the depiction of communities as homogeneous: made up of like-minded people with similar interests.

We now turn to consider more fully the idea of community as a *place*.

2.3   Community as place

The sense of community as a spatially bounded locality, in which relationships are based upon strong personal attachments, was widely used in the late nineteenth century as a critique of the more alienating and less socially cohesive relations which were thought to characterize the rapidly emerging urban-industrial patterns of social life. Traditional modes of living were viewed as more fulfilling and embracing, and community was often regarded in terms which were not only favourable but also idealized and romanticized, and which increasingly relied upon a nostalgia for an imagined past. Here we should note that such appeals to community were an ideological subset within a broader imagined past of an *imagined nation* (see **Lewis, 1998a**).

Notable among the nineteenth-century social theorists who embraced such ideas was the German sociologist Ferdinand Tönnies. Like many of his contemporaries, Tönnies was particularly concerned to offer a sociological interpretation of social change. Writing in the late 1880s, Tönnies (1957) drew a distinction between two types of social organization: *Gemeinschaft* and *Gesellschaft*. While these German terms do not translate directly into English, they have generally been read as 'community' and 'society' respectively. Tönnies distinguished the two types of social organization primarily in terms of the social relations which characterized them. According to Tönnies *Gemeinschaft,* or community, relations are dominated by primary social group bonds, such as those of family and kin, with face-to-face, informal and personalized contact prevailing; *Gesellschaft*-like relations, or those based on society, are dominated by secondary social groups such as work-defined associations and more transitory, anonymous and contractual relationships.

For Tönnies and other social theorists of the period, these contrasting relations were linked with settlement patterns. The 'pre-industrial' rural way of life allowed more immediate and stronger social bonds to develop, with individuals bound by kinship or the soil. Urban-industrial society, on the other hand, was characterized more by secondary, fleeting types of relationships. Thus different kinds of places determined different kinds of social relations. This way of thinking was dominant within urban sociology until the mid-twentieth century (Savage and Warde, 1993). Embedded in anti-urban sentiments, this approach was reflected in a series of attempts to create communities.

From Plato's New Republic through to Thomas More's Utopia in the sixteenth century, new communities have been proposed to solve the perceived social problems of the day. Perhaps the most vivid examples are the 'model communities' actually created in the nineteenth century, for instance, at New Lanark, Bourneville in Birmingham, Saltaire in Bradford and Port Sunlight on

Merseyside. The attempt to create communities resurfaced in the garden city movement in the early twentieth century and in the post-Second World War new town and new housing estate programmes, founded upon an implicit assumption that communities could be socially engineered. What is significant about these developments for our purposes is not whether communities were established, but that the *idea* of community (expressed in the language of 'social mixing', 'neighbourhood units' and 'balanced communities') was important as an ideological device in legitimizing such policies.

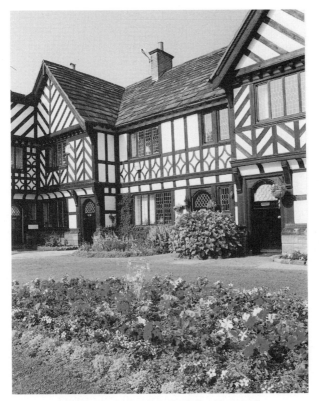

Model community? Port Sunlight, Merseyside

2.3.1 Community studies

Approaches that stressed the golden age of an organic community in some imagined past were questioned by those who drew attention to the prevalence of social divisions, conflicts and widespread inequalities in pre-industrial villages (Sharpe, 1996). Alternative arguments, which appeared to reject the golden age mythology, focused more on the undermining of what were nevertheless viewed as self-sufficient, close-knit communities by processes of industrialization and urbanization, leading to fewer personal ties. But this claim was itself rejected by some of the explorations of working-class life in what has come to be termed the 'community studies' approach of the 1950s and 1960s. The term 'community studies' refers to a series of studies published in the post-war UK which attempted to explore the impact of social change in a variety of locales and social situations (Frankenberg, 1966). Heavily influenced by social anthropology and sociology,

community studies

61

the label 'community studies' does not refer to a coherent school of thought but to a diverse range of research which relied upon different methods and theoretical approaches. Before considering some of the studies and arguments, it is important to consider the wider context within which such studies were conducted.

That the UK was in a state of major change in the aftermath of the Second World War was evident not only in the social sciences, but also in popular literature, the theatre and the cinema. Fictional accounts of life – such as Robert McLeish's *The Gorbals Story* (1946), Allan Sillitoe's *Saturday Night and Sunday Morning* (1958), Shelagh Delaney's *A Taste of Honey* (1958) or *This Sporting Life* by David Storey (1960), as well as popular television dramas such as *Dixon of Dock Green* and *Z-Cars* – took place against a backdrop of social upheaval, with working-class communities under siege from wider processes of economic, industrial, social, moral and demographic change (Laing, 1986).

What is commonly referred to as 'kitchen-sink drama' was a popular means by which novelists and playwrights attempted to grasp and depict the essence of change and its consequences for life in working-class areas. Analysing the lives of the working class had long been a preoccupation of sociology, and during the 1950s and 1960s much of UK sociology in particular was concerned to explore working-class communities amidst the supposedly alienating world of urban-industrialism. This was a world characterized by rapid social change, in which large-scale urban renewal programmes, slum clearance schemes and new town developments wrought major changes in urban areas.

Many of the studies were conducted in either localities dominated by (declining) industries such as coal mining and shipbuilding, or inner-city areas which were seen, in our view problematically, as being disrupted by urban renewal, out-migration and immigration. Other studies concentrated on efforts to establish community in newly created mass housing estates or in the new towns. Two studies in particular characterize much of the research produced at this time.

A generation of young UK sociologists were weaned on what came to be widely regarded as a classic among sociological studies of life in the post-war UK: Young and Willmott's *Family and Kinship in East London*, first published in 1957. Primarily concerned with changes in patterns of family life, this study argued that strong communities had survived the pressures of urbanization, and that in the midst of large-scale urban change there were distinct urban villages with social ties and bonds characteristic of *Gemeinschaft*-like social relations. Bethnal Green, the focus of their study, was considered to have strong kinship links and extended family relations, with a dense complexity of friendship networks. While for Tönnies and his colleagues it was urbanization that had disrupted social life in the nineteenth century, for Young and Willmott, among others, suburbanization and new town development were the culprits. Life in Bethnal Green was very different from that which they claimed was characteristic of the new Greenleigh estate, built to accommodate East London families decanted through slum clearance. In the latter nuclear family ties predominated, there was little sense of a busy community life and the estate lacked the friendliness of Bethnal Green (Young and Willmott, 1957).

According to this account, suburbanization was not simply an exercise in geographical relocation but represented an erosion of an old order and morality. As Lebeau (1997, p.290) commented: 'the journey from Bethnal Green to

Greenleigh is presented as a move from a profoundly familial and recognizable urban space to the "emptiness" of a suburban estate unmarked by memory, thoroughly strange and estranging.'

While family ties were central to the Bethnal Green study, work was seen as a determining characteristic of social life in the second of the community studies which we have chosen to highlight. But, as in Young and Willmott's account, gender divisions were central to the storyline. *Coal is Our Life* (Dennis *et al.*, 1969) was a study of a mining community in Yorkshire in the early 1950s. Dennis and his colleagues argued that little had changed from the inter-war period in terms of values and outlook on life. A highly segregated sexual division of labour characterized the gender relations of the community, while the largely male, paid working environment featured strong feelings of solidarity and trade unionism in opposition to management in general. There was a strong sense of the past, of struggles in years gone by. Patterns of leisure, like employment, were male dominated and reflected the harshness of working conditions, with drinking and rugby league dominating.

These two studies, together with a large number of other accounts of life in the post-war UK, as well as the kitchen-sink dramas, were influential in shaping our senses of what a community is, and in producing what came to be a dominant representation of 'the working-class community' in particular. They also represented a shift from the vision of the organic rural community (in which people of different ranks are bonded to a socially segregated and stratified community). While these studies differed in their methodologies, scope and theoretical stance, they all tended to avoid the issue of how to define 'community'. In his review of community studies in the mid-1960s, Frankenberg (1966, p.15) offered the following definition: 'an area of social living marked by some degree of social coherence. The bases of community are locality and community sentiment.' While this *appears* to offer a concrete and solid definition, problems remain. 'Social coherence', 'locality' and 'community sentiment' are open to a multitude of competing interpretations. In the quest for a workable definition we are, therefore, still left wanting. However, community studies were important in structuring the understanding of community as a bounded place, characterized by certain values, attitudes and patterns of family and working life. But how useful was their depiction of *the* working-class community?

place

These community studies were characterized by certain limitations, albeit to different degrees. In many respects the authors of the various studies were guilty of constructing a stereotypical view of working-class life, one which was at odds with the experience of large sections of the working class in the 1950s and 1960s. The picture of community life presented is largely descriptive and static, ahistorical snapshots of particular aspects of life, for particular groups of people, in particular places at particular moments in time. Besides, a tight-knit, single-class community was not a universal working-class experience. It is also worth noting that the localities depicted as traditionally working class had been forged only during the previous half century or so.

In these studies there is little sense of social *processes*, or dynamic relations between different social groups (Brook and Finn, 1978). For example, while strongly segregated gender roles were a significant feature of Bethnal Green and the Yorkshire mining community, the focus of most of these studies tended to be on the 'male' worlds of work and leisure. The role of female domestic labour was all too often marginalized or completely ignored; women were often invisible in these studies. Steedman (1986, p.16) highlighted the marginalization of some lives and stories in the desire to portray a homogeneous, stable, working-class community. She spoke of her mother who 'ran a working-class household far away from the traditional communities of class, in exile and isolation, and in which a man was not a master, nor even there very much.'

Thus certain relationships and processes were either included or excluded in the dominant representation of community life that emerged in the 1950s and 1960s. Moreover, this representation tended to be characterized by a strong, nostalgic imagery of the past. Bourke (1994, p.169) argued that such communities were 'retrospectively constructed'. By this she means they were the product of both a retrospective and retrograde romanticism of working-class life. Few of the studies drew attention to other aspects of such communities – for example, coercion, domestic violence, sectarianism, racism and sexism. And where the struggle to make ends meet in a world of poverty and deprivation was presented it was often glamorized, for example in the idea of 'turning necessity into a virtue'.

While Young and Willmott were at pains to show that communities remained in large urban centres well into the second half of the twentieth century, they were largely swimming against a tide of popular opinion which argued that community was either in (terminal) decline or had been lost. Thus both the *rediscovery of community* and the *loss of community* are recurring themes in the study of social relationships (among the working class in particular). But, importantly, throughout this period the idea of community never really went away; in fact, the perceived *loss* of community appears to accord the idea a more central place within social discourses.

Community as place, then, forms a key part of the national popular, and the association of community with territory tended to be predominant in many representations of community during the course of the twentieth century. Next we consider some of the ways in which community has been imagined in attempts to avoid the limitations of community as place.

2.4   Community as belonging

ACTIVITY 2.1

The two popular Glaswegian songs below originate in the 1960s and 1970s when Glasgow, like most of the UK's other major cities, was undergoing large-scale redevelopment. Read through each and consider the different ways in which 'traditional' working-class community life is depicted.

THE GLASGOW THAT I USED TO KNOW

Oh, where is the Glasgow where I used tae stey?
The white wally closes done up wi' pipe cley,
where ye knew every neighbour frae first floor tae third,
and to keep your door locked was considered absurd.
Do you know the folk steyin' next door to you?

And where is the wee shop where I used to buy
a quarter o' totties, a tuppenny pie, a bag o' broken
biscuits an three tottie scones; and the wumman aye

asked, 'How's your maw getting on?'
Can your big supermarkets gie service like that?

And where is the wean that wance played in the street.
Wi' a jorrie, a peerie, a gird wi' a cleek?
Can he still cadge a hudgie or dreep off a dyke?
Or is writin' on wa's noo the wan thing he likes?
Can he tell chickie-mellie fae hunch-cuddy-hunch?

And where is the fitba' that I played and saw,
The fair shou'der charge and the pass aff the wa'?
There was nae 4–3–3, there was nae 4–2–4,
And your mates didnae kiss ye whenever ye'd score.
Is the game, like big Woodburn, suspended sine die?

And where is the tramcar that wance did the ton
Up the Great Western Road on the old Yoker run?
The conductress aye knew how to deal wi' a nyaff.
'If ye're gaun then gat oan, if ye're no then get aff!'
Are there ony like her on the buses the day?

And where is the chip-shop that I knew sae well?
The wee corner cafe where they used to sell
Hot peas and brey and Macallums and pokes.
An ye knew they were tallies the minute they spoke:
'Dae ye wanta da raspberry ower yer ice-a-cream?'

Oh where is the Glasgow that I used to know?
Big Wullie, Wee Shooie, the steamie, the Co?
The shilpit wee bauchle, the glaikit big dreep,
The ba' on the slates, and yer gas in a peep?
If ye scrape the veneer aff, are these things still there?

(words by Adam McNaughton, in McVicar, 1990, p.43)

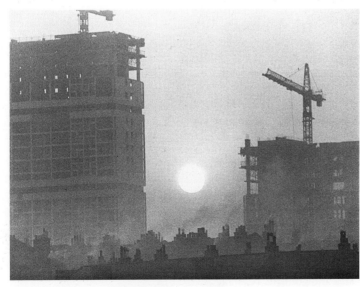

The redevelopment of the Gorbals in the 1960s

FAREWELL TO GLASGOW

Oh where is the Glasgow I used to know?
The tenement buildings that let in the snow.
Through the cracks in the plaster the cold wind did blow,
and the water we washed in was fifty below.

We read by the gaslight, we had nae T.V.,
Hot porridge for breakfast, cold porridge for tea,
Some weans had rickets and some had T.B.,
Aye, that's what the Glasgow of old means to me.

Noo the neighbours complained if we played wi'a ba',
Or hunch-cuddy-hunch against somebody's wa',
If we played kick-the-can we'd tae watch for the law,
And the polis made sure we did sweet bugger a'.

And we huddled together to keep warm in bed,
We had nae sheets or blankets, just auld coats instead,
And a big balaclava to cover your head,
and 'God, but it's cold' was the only prayer said.

Noo there's some say that tenement living was swell,
That's the wally-close toffs who had doors wi' a bell,
Two rooms and a kitchen and a bathroom as well,
While the rest of us lived in a single-end hell.

So wipe aff that smile when you talk o' the days
Ye lived in the Gorbals or Cowcaddens ways.
Remember the rats and the mice ye once chased.
For tenement living was a bloody disgrace.

(words and music by Jim McLean, in McVicar, 1990, p. 91)

COMMENT

In *The Glasgow That I Used to Know* McNaughton depicts a rather romanticized view of Glasgow's tenement life. What comes across strongly is a sense of closeness and togetherness: everyone knew everyone else and there was a sense of communality. It was a world of small corner shops giving good service, where football was alive and spontaneous. McLean's *Farewell to Glasgow* was written partly as a critical response to McNaughton's song. Here tenement living is more harshly depicted, with poor quality housing, ill-health and a host of deprivations strongly featured. McLean also draws attention to the divide between good quality tenement houses where 'toffs' lived and rat-infested, slum-ridden working-class homes.

These two songs carry contested stories. It is not the case that either McNaughton or McLean are right or wrong. As Barnes (1997, p.5) noted, there is no one truth about what community is. Both songwriters provide particular representations of life in Glasgow's tenement districts.

Both songs share a strong sense of class belonging and, albeit implicitly, feelings of class conflict and class antagonism. (The idea of community is all too often deployed in ways that, despite references to 'working-class communities', obscure class relations and class antagonisms (Callinicos, 1996).)

The Glasgow songs, and others like them, are just some of the ways in which community has been constructed as a sense of belonging. In many respects this is the most popular way in which community is imagined, but again we would emphasize that this overlaps with other ideas of community. In constructing community as a sense of belonging, or belongings, we start to question the idea of community as a place-bounded phenomenon, as well as some of the more conservative interpretations of traditional communities.

belonging

■ ■ ■

2.5   Rethinking community

Williams (1988) observed that community is a 'warmly persuasive word' which never seems to be used unfavourably. But increasingly this is no longer the case. A number of social scientists and political activists have drawn attention to the more oppressive side of community and have suggested that we need to rethink community, avoiding the emotive value judgements that have plagued the idea. In rethinking the notion of community we need to unpack some of its more hidden meanings, as well as its implications for social policy analysis. To begin this we need to consider the limitations of the uses of community discussed above.

The idea that community refers to a spatially bounded locality is problematic. It tends to suggest that there is something natural, permanent and exclusive about such a place; that it is separate and distinct from other places. In the process, internal divisions, conflicts and struggles are all too often neglected in the desire to project communities as harmonious and homogeneous. A number of critics have drawn attention to the ways in which people and places are always connected with others (Gilroy, 1997). Communities of identity can be created out of local–global links. Thus Eade (1997) argued that globalization does not inevitably destroy identities but can lead to the creation of new hybrid communities, through, for example, patterns of migration. 'Globalization' is the term used to describe the trend by which events, decisions and activities in one part of the globe come to have increasingly significant consequences for people and localities in quite distant parts of the world (McGrew, 1992). Local communal solidarities, for example among Bangladeshis in London's East End or the Irish in Manchester or Glasgow, owe as much to (past and present) global processes as to more localized relations. In this sense, then, there is a struggle *for* community, that is, a struggle to maintain or make communities. To take a different example, for New World Africans music has been of signal importance in forging communities from the uprooted histories of their dispersal. The recognition that community can be forged in ways dissociated from place is useful in rethinking community.

Are communities in the dominant senses we have traditionally attached to them desirable? Young (1990) rejects this claim by arguing that the privilege given to face-to-face, small-scale relations is misplaced. In the traditional sense of community, the recognition of difference and diversity is repressed. For Young, and other critics such as Sennett (1996), this repression lies at the centre of the dangers of community.

We have already noted that the stereotypical representation of working-class communities played down the significance of gender divisions. In the late

1960s, for example, this was a feature of the reports of the National Community Development Projects in the UK. These state-managed, localized anti-poverty programmes tended to deny the significance of such divisions in their portrayal of homogeneous working-class communities (Green and Chapman, 1992). It is important, therefore, that we see community in its traditional guise(s) as fundamentally gendered, and as racialized.

As we have seen, because of its elasticity and the overwhelmingly positive attributes attached to it, the term 'community' is often used simply as a descriptor of certain aspects of social life. But it is argued here that community also legitimizes certain relations and critiques others. This is evident when we consider the ways in which community has tended to be embedded in a particular expression of gender relations.

ACTIVITY 2.2

Read the following comments from Tony Blair and John Major. As you read them consider what sense of community they are using. In what ways is community linked with representations of the family?

> I have no doubt that the breakdown of law and order is intimately linked to the break-up of a strong sense of community. And the break-up of community in turn is, to a crucial degree, consequent on the breakdown in family life. If we want anything more than a superficial discussion on crime and its causes, we cannot ignore the importance of the family.
>
> (Tony Blair speaking in the aftermath of the Jamie Bulger murder, quoted in Callinicos, 1996, p.16)

> History will call it the Decent Society, a new social order for the Age of Achievement for Britain. We will respect family life, develop it in any way we can because strong families are the foundation of strong communities.
>
> (Tony Blair, speech to the Labour Party Conference, 1996)

> [T]he long shadows falling across the county ground, the warm beer, the invincible green suburbs, dog lovers and pools fillers ... old maids bicycling to Holy Communion though the morning mist.
>
> (John Major recalling the England of his childhood in his St George's Day Speech, 1993)

COMMENT

Blair makes direct links between community and family. This is not a new departure by any means; the two concepts are often treated together and are equally contested and elusive. They are commonly constructed as 'naturalness'. Linking social relationships such as community with familial ones can provide them with a powerful reinforcement (Weeks, 1991), and indeed the gendered ideology of familialism is at the heart of many representations of community. For Blair the decline in community is associated directly with family breakdown, leading to increasing moral decay and social disorganization. Such claims are not far removed from arguments that a new socially excluded underclass has emerged in the UK in the latter stages of the twentieth century (**Morris, 1998**).

Smith (1997, p.183) has argued that family and community have become central to the Labour Party's political discourse. Exhortations to return to family values and to rebuild communities, she claims, are an attempt to address the growing problem of poverty, especially among younger families, and increasing social disintegration in poor communities, but without additional financial resources from central government.

Major presents a fondly held image of the village in 'middle England'. Taken together these quotations imply nostalgia and positive feelings for community. But they also imply a critique of (certain aspects) of modernity by suggesting the naturalness of community, distinct gender roles and family life, premised upon a particular understanding and representation of gender and class relations.

■ ■ ■

Community can be the locale of much of women's oppression, where stifling meanings of masculinity and femininity are enforced. But it can also be a source of support and collective solidarity. In this sense, community is contradictory. Williams (1993) argued that community can mean different things to different women. On the one hand, community as *space* allows for the struggle for representation, the struggle to make hidden voices heard, for better housing, crèche provision or health facilities. Thus, in the 1984–85 miners' strike, community-based women's groups were instrumental not only in supporting the strikers, but also in pushing the boundaries of women's position within coalfield communities and beyond, challenging the rigid domestic division of labour (Beaton, 1985; Stead, 1987). On the other hand, community can be the place in which women are confined. The idea of community as *place* implies a rigid sexual division of labour, where social welfare in general, and community caring in particular, can be done at little or no cost to anyone except the predominantly female workers who have to supply it.

This distinction between community as space and community as place helps us to grasp the contradictions within, and some of the different meanings accorded to, community. Community emerges here as a source both of constraint and as a source of social support to be fought for.

Southall Black Sisters, a group of Asian and African-Caribbean women founded in 1979 in Southall, London, struggled against a sense of community that effectively ignored domestic violence and sexual harassment (Southall Black Sisters, 1989). Southall has long been demonized as a problem locale, particularly in relation to 'racial' tensions. It was the people of Southall who rallied so effectively against the National Front in 1979. Against both the internal and external representation of Southall as a homogeneous community, the Southall Black Sisters argued that it was deeply divided. They challenged views of community in which certain interests were allowed to dominate and be articulated as the interests of the *whole* community. Like the Women Against Pit Closures movement in the mid 1980s, they sought to construct new senses of belonging which recognized the multi-layered nature of everyday experiences in which both racism and sexism featured strongly. This, then, was an attempt to forge an idea of community that recognized different senses of belonging.

One of the central points to emerge thus far is that we need to reject much of the imagery, romanticism and exclusiveness which has been a dominant feature of writings about community. We also need to repudiate the idea that communities are in some sense natural, that boundaries between social groups of people, and between places, are permanent and static. Communities are, above all, socially constructed.

Community should not be seen as a once and for all entity; people can shift in and out of different communities at different times, and may occupy a number of overlapping communities at any one time. As a result of this they may experience conflicting identities (Charles and Davies, 1997, p.419). Communities may also contain internal divisions. In other words, communities will always be plural and overlapping. They are formed, made and struggled for and over.

But if we accept that communities are more dynamic than the dominant representations, and reject the simple analysis of an idealized golden past, does this mean that there are no boundaries between communities, that membership is open with no exclusions, and that there is now a greater acceptance of other communities?

Bellos (1997) argues that the increasing diversity and complexity of modern life is reflected in new types of community, communities of identity and alternative communities. Thus community appears again as a seductive way of imagining new belongings and connections. In rejecting the formula that communities of place are necessarily communities of (common) interest(s), we decouple the idea of community from a sense of place. Non-place forms of community and identity have been forged or are in the process of being formed (see, for example, Weeks, 1996). Thus we can rather easily accept that there are multiple communities, that there is diversity, but the question of who belongs to which community/ies remains.

Gilroy (1987, p.235) argued that community is as much about difference as it is about similarity and identity. It is about boundaries, struggles, conflicts. It is, fundamentally, a relational idea. Thus boundaries remain a necessary feature of communities. These may in part be physical as in, for example, the emergence of fortress or gated communities in major cities in the USA (Davis, 1990; Christophersen, 1994), but they are also shaped by ideas of who should be included and excluded. Thus community can still be seen as potentially marginalizing, premised as it is upon the exclusion of 'others'; the recognition of diversity does not in itself mean that inequalities and exclusions are challenged and contested.

When the notion of a British community is utilized, who belongs and what images are used?

The notion of a British community invariably implies 'the indigenous', where certain sentiments and customs are shared, where there are insiders and outsiders. But other communities may not share this collective sentiment. Do immigrants (and who are 'immigrants'?) form part of this community? What about the Irish in Britain, or the Scots or the Welsh? Are socially excluded and marginalized 'welfare ghetto' estates part of this national community? They clearly appear to be excluded from the dominant images of such a community. In many respects such localities form part of an imagined 'other' against which one type of community can be projected. These 'excluded' localities are often portrayed as lacking community cohesion, characterized by community 'pathology'. However, some localities are constructed as not fitting in because they have *too much* community (such as South Asian groups). Indeed it is the perceived absence of community, or of an overbearingly self-contained 'alien' community, that has led some proponents of communitarianism to argue that unless such communities are brought into the 'wider community' the consequences for social cohesion may be dire. The stigmatization of such

London Docklands: reimagining community?

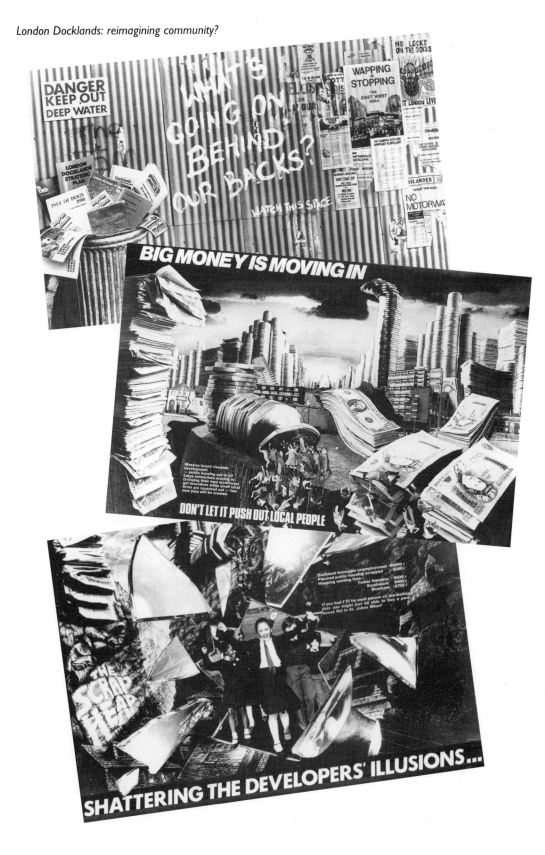

localities as lacking community is often at odds with those who live there. In a major study of life in Manchester and Sheffield, Taylor and his colleagues commented that:

> there was widespread consensus about the existence and identity of a number of undesirable problem estates in each city, but also an impressive level of agreement about the distinct advantages and qualities of others ... Even in the case of the most demonized estates of all, we found ... people ... who wanted to speak well of the strong sense of community and neighbourliness that could be found there.
>
> (Taylor *et al.*, 1996, p.296)

Here, community is deployed as a way of capturing everyday connections and relations. In notions and representations of community, inequalities and ideas of class, gender, 'race', age, sexuality, etc. are ever present, but in ways that render their presence invisible. Community may appear as a progressive symbolic figure through which some social relationships can be *reimagined*, but we need to continually question the assumptions, and the social divisions upon which this is based.

Where does this take us with the notion of community? Not with a clearer sense of definition, certainly, but with an increased awareness of the contested, ambiguous and contradictory nature of community. Community is symbolic; it appears almost as magical. Communities are always *imagined* (Anderson, 1983). Perhaps they exist as a necessary fiction, through which attempts are made to make sense of the world; whereby links are forged and through which mobilization and resistance to marginalization and exclusions can be conducted. But alongside the awareness of diversity and differentiation, ideas of community continue to have a deeply moral resonance. Community is a fundamentally political concept. As such it is 'saturated with power' (Hoggett, 1997, p.14). This will become evident in our discussions of moral communitarianism and radical left pluralism in section 3.

In this section we have explored in some depth the conceptual complexities surrounding the idea of community. In particular we have focused on the ways in which sociologists have analysed the problem of speaking of community in the singular and as something necessarily rooted in a specific locality. For all its ambiguities and slipperiness, it is clear that appeals to community retain a powerful resonance in both popular and policy discourses about the future of welfare. This resonance is at its most powerful in the contemporary welfare discourse around community care. In the next section we explore how the debate about being a member of a community (or, less commonly, communit*ies*) has come to the fore in the new politics of welfare. In particular we explore the extent to which the appeal to community membership may represent an important and contested attempt to construct new subjects of social welfare.

3 Two contrasting appeals to community for a welfare future

3.1 Introduction

This section focuses on two broad, contrasting and opposed uses of community as a means of realizing a more cohesive social welfare order in the future: moral communitarianism and radical left pluralism.

Whereas section 2 introduced you to the subtle and highly nuanced conceptual distinctions raised by social scientific analyses of the meanings of community, the aim, and thus the tone, of this section is somewhat different. Here you will be required to evaluate two quite starkly opposed ideological, moral and political discourses around the politics of community and possible futures of welfare. You will be confronted, therefore, with a debate between two groups of protagonists about the contested nature of community and welfare in contemporary society. The contributions that we present in this section may be said to be closer to political pamphleteering than 'detached' social science. Put simply, pamphleteering may be described as the production by intellectuals of moral and political discourses. It was an important activity of intellectuals in Britain and Ireland throughout the eighteenth and nineteenth centuries and, unlike much academic social scientific writing which is largely aimed at an academic audience, pamphleteering is aimed at a public or popular audience.

pamphleteering

We begin by presenting an exposition, or descriptive outline, of the two opposed intellectual positions on community. A brief critique of each will then help you to reach your own conclusions about the relative merits and limitations of each position as a means of imagining both a new welfare settlement and the recasting of the national popular.

ACTIVITY 2.3

Section 3.2 outlines the arguments presented by four proponents of moral communitarianism: Amitai Etzioni, Norman Dennis, Melanie Phillips and David Green. As you read these outlines you should note the main arguments and your own criticisms of them. You will use these notes in Activity 2.7.

You may find it useful to use a grid such as this for your notes.

	Main arguments	Critique of arguments
Etzioni		
Dennis		
Phillips		
Green		

3.2 The moral communitarian appeal to the community as the basis for the remoralization of society

We begin this section by introducing you to the philosophical roots and key themes of the communitarian critique of contemporary society. The moral communitarian appeal to the community as the basis for the remoralization of society and a new welfare order is then explored in some depth through the writings of four conservative commentators. We begin with Etzioni's popular manifesto of moral communitarianism which emerged in the 1990s in the USA. We then examine the conservative, moralizing discourse in the UK around community as 'the new common sense'. This is especially associated with the pamphleteering work of Dennis, Phillips, and Green and the Institute of Economic Affairs, the neo-conservative think-tank. The next section provides a critique of moral communitarianism.

3.2.1 The philosophical roots of communitarianism

The word 'communitarianism' may be new to you. In the UK and the USA during the 1990s it became a popular and influential way of describing political and ideological appeals to community values and common moral virtues, in reaction to the apparent decline in civic morality and growth in individualism and welfare

moral communitarian dependency. More specifically, moral communitarian thought claims to reject the market-led ideology of the New Right, the liberal/libertarian emphasis on individual rights, and the top-down approach to welfare from the state.

The intellectual and philosophical roots of communitarianism are decidedly mixed. As well as important connections back to Aristotelian notions of civic republicanism and Judaeo-Christian ideas of communion, the expression of communitarian aspirations is associated with the radical thought of the early utopian socialists and anarchists such as Robert Owen and Peter Kropotkin. Furthermore, communitarian philosophy may also be linked to the conservative sociological tradition associated with Tönnies (see section 2.3) and, to a lesser extent, Emile Durkheim. As a body of thought communitarianism appears to be neither *for* the state nor *for* the individual. Lasch (1995, p.101), for example, noted that it is difficult to classify communitarianism on the conventional spectrum of political opinion. Thus, for example, within communitarian thought the extremes of both the market and the state are viewed as dangers to the vibrant, organic, welfare community, and liberalism's emphasis on individual rights and abstract notions of enlightened self-interest is criticized for its neglect of the inherently social nature of humans and the collective character of human existence.

The philosopher Alisdair MacIntyre (1981) offers us the clearest statement of moral communitarian ideas about the relationship between the individual and society. MacIntyre is at odds with the liberal tradition of political thought epitomized by the work of John Rawls. Rawls's (1973) thesis, put simply, is that if, hypothetically, individuals knew nothing about their position in society – their wealth, their abilities, their life-chances or their welfare needs – they would agree with one another that they should live in a society in which everyone enjoyed the greatest measure of freedom compatible with that of others. In turn, inequalities would be tolerated only in so far as the results benefited the least well placed. Here, then, we have a view of society/community as being based on a contract between calculating and free individuals. Against this thesis of a rational social contract, MacIntyre argues that we cannot help but know about our position in society and that we are not atomized, isolated individuals but essentially social beings, rooted in real families and communities. He views the stress on individual freedom in liberal political thought as being over-played. However, MacIntyre is not optimistic about what can be done about the lack of common morals in modern societies. He suggests that because of the decline in common moral values in individualistic capitalist societies we are no longer able to decide between rival moral views. To find the 'answer' to the malaise of modern societies, MacIntyre looks back to ancient Greek society and the philosophical thought of Aristotle. In particular, Aristotle argued for the importance of individuals being firmly located in a coherent ethical tradition which recommended ways of being and acting, 'virtues' which in turn were firmly based in concrete forms of social life.

For MacIntyre, a person is fully human only when she or he is part of a coherent communal tradition, since it is through a tradition that an individual gains self-understanding, and through concrete social practices established by that tradition that she of he is able to live a meaningful life. Through the tradition to which we belong, we are able to cast ourselves as a character in the life of our community and thus adopt a life-plan. In MacIntyre's (1981, p.203) words, 'I inherit from the past of my family, my city, my tribe, my nation, a variety of debts, inheritances, rightful expectations and obligations. These constitute the given of my life, my moral starting point.'

A brief summary of this debate between liberal political theorists and their communitarian critics highlights the political and ideological appeal of the moral communitarian discourse for politicians and policy-makers in the post-welfare state. According to liberal political theorists the moral sovereignty of the individual is the first principle from which to start (see Chapter 1 on the 'consumer'). They therefore stress the importance of adopting political institutions that uphold this principle. In contrast, both conservative and radical communitarian thinkers argue that society and the socialization of its members are logically and factually a precondition of individuals. Therefore, all social arrangements – including the provision and delivery of social welfare – are best understood (and all policies best pursued) as attempts to make individuals aware of their common interests in co-operation.

As Jordan (1996, pp.20–1) notes, this intellectual debate entered the practical welfare politics of the 1990s as governments sought to soften conflicts, promote consensus, produce trust and obedience to rules and encourage identification with fellow citizens. Given that there appeared to be little support for the strategy of trying to restore harmony and collective social welfare through the redistribution of wealth and increased state benefits and services on the lines of the Beveridgean welfare settlement (see **Hughes, 1998**), there was an urgent concern among modern states to find a new cement or glue for society. The communitarian appeal to the community was thus attractive across the political spectrum. As Bowring (1997, p.93) noted, the importance of a widespread sense of social or communal membership to the healthy functioning of modern society is now rarely disputed. The popular political appeal of the communitarian discourse is therefore unsurprising.

Communitarianism:
the new super-glue?

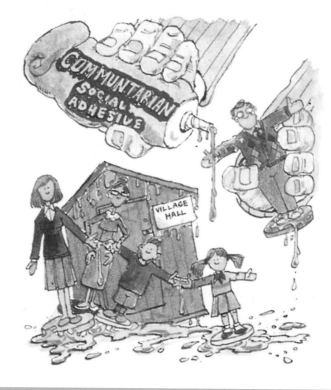

ACTIVITY 2.4

Read the following statements from Lasch and Braithwaite, which convey the broad drift of the communitarian tradition. In particular try to answer the following questions:

1   What do Lasch and Braithwaite argue is the basis of social order and welfare in human societies?

2   What might be implied from these statements about the balance between individual rights and collective duties in communitarian thinking?

> Communitarianism … found the sources of social cohesion in shared assumptions so deeply engrained in everyday life that they do not have to be articulated: in folkways, customs, prejudices, habits of the heart.
>
> (Lasch, 1995, p.92)

> In communitarian societies individuals are densely enmeshed in inter-dependencies which have special qualities of mutual help and trust. The interdependencies have symbolic significance in the culture of group loyalties which take precedence over individual interests.
>
> (Braithwaite, 1989, p.100)

COMMENT

Much of the appeal of communitarianism is to 'real' people in specific, bounded communities rather than to the abstract notions of liberty and individual rights of liberalism. Much of our welfare needs will thus depend on our close relations and interdependencies with members of our 'in group'. Because of this we may note the strong conservative appeal of communitarianism, implying notions of exclusive group membership and long-established traditions, or what Lasch terms 'habits of the heart'. Furthermore, both social order and social welfare are seen as being maintained principally on the basis of informal social mechanisms within communities of interdependent members (which, as we saw in section 2, are often profoundly gendered). Obligation and duty to the group would appear to count for more than individual rights. A strong and recurrent emphasis is placed by all communitarians on duties and responsibilities to the wider civil society rather than freedoms and rights for the individual. Social compliance in turn derives primarily from informal controls built into everyday relations.

■ ■ ■

3.2.2 'Born in the USA': Etzioni's moral communitarian manifesto

The most populist moral communitarian commentator in the 1990s was the American sociologist Amitai Etzioni. The context for his critique of US society (and by implication other modern societies such the UK), and his manifesto for the remoralization of society, is a USA which has been viewed as the most powerful and most extreme capitalist society in terms of its celebration and institutionalization of the free market, the individual and materialism. The following quotation represents the kernel of Etzioni's self-consciously simple message: 'Communitarians call to restore civic virtues, for people to live up to their responsibilities and not to merely focus on their entitlements, and to shore up the moral foundations of society' (Etzioni, 1995, p.ix).

In the preface to the first UK edition of *The Spirit of Community*, Etzioni pointed out that the expression of communitarian ideas was increasingly to be found in politicians of diverse political persuasions in the USA, the UK and mainland Europe. Etzioni's explanation for influential politicians getting on board the communitarian platform, and thereby apparently breaking the mould of traditional party and ideological positions, is quite simple: 'they are visionary people who have seen the power of a compelling set of ideas whose time has come' (1995, p.ix). Such claims to influencing politicians are acknowledged even by the critics of Etzioni's communitarian manifesto. Accordingly, Bowring (1997, p.98) noted that Etzioni's work 'has provided a fertile vocabulary for policy-makers and politicians in Britain, many of whom recognize his fear of society's moral decline – and the more political of whom know this anxiety is a potential source of electoral support.'

In the following passage Etzioni presents his manifesto for communitarianism in terms of it offering the middle way between the two extremes of 'authoritarians' and 'radical individualists':

> We adopted the name *Communitarian* to emphasize that the time had come to attend to our responsibilities to the conditions and elements we all share, to the community.
>
> As Communitarians we also recognized a need for a new social, philosophical, and political map. The designation of political camps as liberals or conservatives, as left or right, often no longer serves. We see at one extreme Authoritarians ... They urge the imposition on all others of moral positions they believe in, from prayer in schools to forcing women to stay in the kitchen. At the other end we see Radical Individualists ... who believe that if individuals are left on their own to pursue their choices, rights, and self-interests, all will be well. We suggest that *free individuals require a community*, which backs them up against encroachment by the state and sustains

morality by drawing on the gentle prodding of kin, friends, neighbors, and other community members, rather than building on government controls or fear of authorities.

(Etzioni, 1995, p.15)

What are the main themes conveyed by Etzioni in his description of communitarianism?

As a self-proclaimed social movement, Etzioni's communitarianism seeks the regeneration of *moral obligation* between citizens. More specifically, Etzioni's (1994) manifesto focuses on three interrelated areas of concern:

1   the shoring up of morality in civil institutions such as the family, school and voluntary associations;

2   the addressing and reversal of the problem of 'too many rights, too few obligations';

3   the assertion of the importance of the public interest as against special interests in political life.

In *The Spirit of Community: The Reinvention of American Society*, Etzioni produced a manifesto that brims over with evidence drawing on a mix of simple moral tales, social scientific data and anecdotal material. This evidence is used to support a call for Americans to face up to their 'responsibilities and duties' to the moral consensus, though the call is always qualified by a concern to avoid any accusation of discrimination against minorities, unless they are 'dangerous and criminal'. However, at times Etzioni (1994, p.22) is quite explicit in harking back to a more stable, orderly and lawful past in the 1950s when 'most Americans spoke with one voice.' In this possibly romanticized view of the past, there is a clear vision of community as a sense of belonging and security, and we are left to ponder who were the other, the 'not most' Americans. Etzioni expresses concern that the previous bedrock of moral consensus has not been replaced by anything of substance other than 'a strong sense of entitlement and a weak sense of obligation', and that this has resulted in an extremely self-centred outlook, or what Etzioni (1994, p.3, p.27) terms a 'me-istic orientation' associated with the libertarian individualism of the 1980s. Furthermore, this rights-based, 'me-istic orientation' is viewed as carrying morally hazardous as well as economically costly welfare consequences by both creating a welfare state dependency culture and undermining communities' capacity for voluntary self-help and succour.

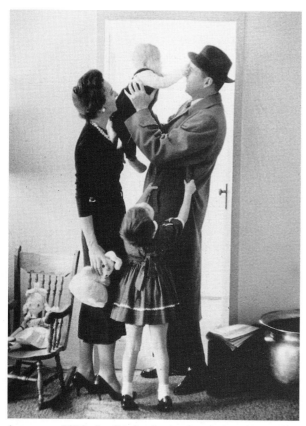

A return to 1950s family values?

In Extract 2.1 Etzioni argues that the balance between rights and obligations in the late twentieth-century USA had become dangerously skewed towards rights and away from duties. As you read the extract focus on the following question: what does Etzioni see as offering the solution to the moral malaise in late twentieth-century US society with particular reference to social welfare?

Extract 2.1 Etzioni: 'The spirit of community'

From time to time there's a finding of social science that may by itself be of limited importance but illuminates a major conundrum. A study has shown that young Americans expect to be tried before a jury of their peers but are rather reluctant to serve on one. This paradox highlights a major aspect of contemporary American civic culture: a strong sense of entitlement – that is, a demand that the community provide more services and strongly uphold rights – coupled with a rather weak sense of obligation to the local and national community. Thus, most Americans applauded the show of force in Grenada, Panama, and in the Persian Gulf, but many were reluctant to serve in the armed forces or see their sons and daughters called up …

Even if lawyers and judges realize among themselves that individual rights are limited by the rights of others and the needs of the community, as the language of rights penetrates into everyday discourse, the discourse becomes impoverished and confrontational. It is one thing to claim that you and I have different interests and see if we can work out a compromise; or, better yet, that we both recognize the merit or virtue of a common cause, say, a cleaner environment. The moment, however, that I claim a *right* to the same piece of land or property or public space as you, we start to view one another like the Catholics and Protestants in Northern Ireland or the Palestinians and Israelis in the Middle East.

A return to a language of social virtues, interests, and, above all, social responsibilities will reduce contentiousness and enhance social cooperation …

To take and not to give is an amoral, self-centred predisposition that ultimately no society can tolerate. To revisit the finding that many try to evade serving on a jury, which, they claim, they have a right to be served by, is egotistical, indecent, and in the long run impractical. Hence, *those most concerned about rights ought to be the first ones to argue for the resumption of responsibilities*. One presumes the other. Much of the following discussion about the conditions under which moral commitments can be strengthened in the family, schools, and in communities speaks directly to the shoring up of our responsibilities. Indeed, many of our core values entail concern for others and the commons we share. As we restore the moral voice of communities (and the web of social bonds, the communitarian nexus, that enables us to speak as a community), we shall see, we will also be more able to encourage one another to live up to our social responsibilities.

(Etzioni, 1994, pp.7, 9–10)

Etzioni contends that in the late twentieth century there was too much emphasis on individual entitlements or rights (delivered through the state) and not enough attention paid to civic obligations to others. The welfare solution which Etzioni offers appears to lie at the level of morals and, in particular, social responsibilities, with communities, especially through the family and schools, given back their moral voice to encourage all their members to act virtuously. All this is in sharp contrast to both the centralized top-down organization of welfare associated with the post-war welfare state and the self-centred rights orientation of liberalism. Etzioni argues that the broad challenge facing countries such as USA and the UK is the 'remoralization' of society, in contrast to the 'de-moralization' associated with individualism at the end of the twentieth century. (On the parallels with nineteenth-century philanthropic concerns over de-moralization of 'the masses', see **Mooney, 1998**).

remoralization

■ ■ ■

With regard to practical welfare policy, the thesis of a 'parenting deficit', particularly among the supposed underclass (see **Morris, 1998**), is to the fore in Etzioni's work, although he is careful to state that this deficit concerns both men and women as parents, and that they should receive support from what Etzioni (1994, p.55) vaguely refers to as the 'wider community' and state. The parenting deficit thesis suggests that, compared to previous decades, the needs of children were not being well attended to in the last decades of the twentieth century. Etzioni (1994, p.70) is in no doubt that delinquency is a reflection of the home from which the young people come. Modern parents are viewed as falling down on their responsibilities to children due to such phenomena as family breakdown, working excessive hours, the 'me-istic' orientation and welfare (state) dependency. Etzioni argues that marriage, in particular, should be awarded more status in a pro-family policy, as the prime expression of our civil responsibilities. At the level of concrete welfare policy, then, Etzioni's brand of communitarianism places a premium on familial parenting and would actively discourage parents from splitting up; dissuade single women from having children; support generous maternity and paternity leave; and improve child-care facilities to make it easier for one parent to stay at home. The following statement captures his position on parenting:

> These ideas about the need to restore our sense of community supersede the left–right political debate. When I'm attacked by both sides I know I'm in the right place. On the family the left tends to say that anything goes. The right wants to put women back in the nursery. They are both wrong. The core of our whole movement is that we hold that fathers and mothers have the same duties and the same rights, and should stay together until the children are grown. We owe that to our children, to ourselves for the civilising experience of parenting, and to the wider society which has a right to expect its new members to be raised responsibly.
>
> (Etzioni, quoted in *The Guardian*, 1995, p.10)

Underpinning Etzioni's analysis of the specific ills of the USA is the recurrent theme of a collapse of a common moral base, beginning in the family and then spreading through the wider community. This close connection between community and family was highlighted in section 2.4, and we return to it below.

Etzioni puts forward quite specific suggestions on law and order which further reinforce the dominant motif of placing obligations on to the community, and the shoring up of 'our' moral foundations, above individual rights. Apart from support for community policing and neighbourhood watch schemes, Etzioni's law and order agenda appears to lend support to a draconian version of 'reintegrative public shaming' (Hughes, 1996). Thus, for first offenders only, Etzioni (1994, p.141) supports a strategy of public humiliation which allows community reintegration, as it would 'serve to underscore society's disapproval of the crime committed rather than of the people themselves. Temporarily marking out those convicted in open court, after due process, seems a legitimate community-building device.' The bottom line for Etzioni in the fight against crime and disorder appears to be the existence of a tight and homogeneous moral community. Thus he argues that the level of crime is deeply affected by the total communal fabric, and he cites the state of Utah as an exemplary oasis of order and low criminality in the USA in the late twentieth century, 'where families are strong, schools teach moral values, communities are well intact, and values command respect' (1994, p.190). Here we may note the attraction of such ideas to politicians from all the major parties in the UK in the 1990s (Hughes, 1996).

Etzioni's moral communitarianism appeared to touch a widespread concern over the effects of both what may be termed marketized individualism and the notion that it was possible to base society on the consumer's right of choice in the market place (see Chapter 1), as well as the expensive 'dependency culture' of state-based welfare. It has also influenced an important body of neo-conservative social commentary in the UK during the late 1990s.

3.2.3 Community as the new common sense in the UK: the work of Dennis, Phillips and Green

Dennis on fatherless families

The work of Norman Dennis focuses on the threat to moral order from what he termed state welfare-dependent 'fatherless families' in the UK in the last decades of the twentieth century. At the core of Dennis's work on families and social problems is the thesis that the monogamous heterosexual family is the crucial and natural unit of social stability in all human societies, and thus the vital means of controlling disorder and delivering social welfare (Dennis, 1993; 1997; Dennis and Erdos, 1993). Dennis further contends that the stable family has been weakened by the permissive, 'me, me' culture promulgated by 'radical libertarian' intellectuals since the 1960s. Radical libertarianism is seen by Dennis as being the leftist intellectual orthodoxy which questions and thus undermines traditional values (such as respect for authority and duty to serve others). Furthermore, radical libertarian intellectuals are accused of promoting an egoistic emphasis on individual freedoms and rights.

For Dennis, this libertarian culture has created a dramatic moral weakening in the most vulnerable sections of society, namely the lower working class, which has become a welfare-dependent underclass. Dennis claims to speak to common sense, and thus to the ordinary 'man', in his self-conscious use of jargon-free language and his appeals to 'natural' explanations of contemporary social problems. He claims to show that children of unmarried single parents do less well on a whole number of fronts than do the offspring of married couples. In particular, he argues that young males from lone mother and state welfare-dependent households are turning to crime and incivilities in increasing numbers due to the loss of positive and disciplining male role models. As the American social commentator Charles Murray (1996, p.127) argued: 'in communities without fathers, the kids tend to run wild' (see **Morris, 1998**).

Dennis is careful not to blame the rising crime rate and the breakdown in law and order on poverty and unemployment. Instead, he sees the roots of rising crime as lying in the abandonment of proper moral standards regarding marriage and, in particular, the activities of conceiving and rearing children.

common sense

Again, Dennis's thesis echoes the view of Murray (1996, p.133) that 'young men are essentially barbarians for whom marriage … is an indispensable civilizing force.' Accordingly, Dennis (1993, p.7) bemoans the fact that the project of creating and maintaining the skills and motivations of fatherhood was being abandoned in the UK during the last decades of the twentieth century, not least as a result of the heritage of the welfare state. We shall see later that it may be argued that there is a distinctive (and conservative) view of human nature underlying both Dennis's specific argument about families and the moral communitarian discourse generally.

In accord with Etzioni, Dennis points to the dangerous loss of both social cohesion and self-control which occurred during and after the 1960s, in contrast to the halcyon days of Dennis's hometown of Sunderland in the 1930s, when there was community and when 'social control was pervasive and consensual, and therefore low-key, good-natured and effective' (Dennis and Erdos, 1993, p.21). The basis of both social order and social welfare is thus taken to reside in the informal mechanisms of civil society and the family rather than in the interventions of the (welfare) state.

> In non-authoritarian societies – 'free' in the sense that social order depends upon self-control rather than control by the agents of the State – crimes increase to the extent that the mechanisms of socialization and the mores lose their ability to reproduce and maintain a culture of decent mutual respect, trust, and restraint.
>
> (Dennis and Erdos, 1993, p.84–5)

'Some mothers do 'ave 'em': the 'old' working-class community

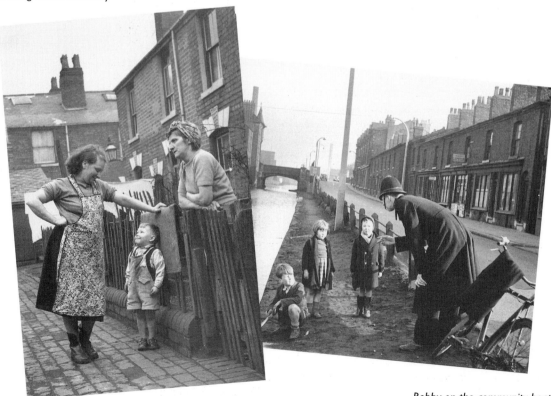

Bobby on the community beat

Phillips on the 'No blame, no shame, no pain society'

In *All Must Have Prizes*, Melanie Phillips, a popular 1990s commentator and journalist, offered a critique of the excessive individualism which she argued swept through the UK during and after the 1960s, causing the greatest damage to children because of what she termed 'the flight from parenting' (Phillips, 1996, p.233). Looking back at the 1970s and 1980s, Phillips presented the following diagnosis of the moral crisis of the family:

> The family had been redefined as the sum of individual decisions uprooted from tradition, custom or obligation. It was a short step from the new short-term contract culture of marriage to regarding the family as just another consumer choice among many. If there are no binding obligations, if commitment is infinitely negotiable, then individuals are free to shop around for sexual partners with whom they may make arrangements to suit their particular circumstances. Within the family itself, children themselves came to be seen as merely products.
>
> (Phillips, 1996, pp.258–9)

Phillips, like Dennis and Etzioni, makes a powerful argument for the close relationship between family breakdown and community decline and, in turn, the growth of social problems among young people. The following quotation sums up Phillips's moral communitarian thesis on the primacy of family-based collective duties over individual rights:

> The causes of disorder are highly complex and difficult to disentangle from each other. But it appears clear that the roots of crime lie in a breakdown of the moral sense which occurs in certain circumstances, leading to a collapse of both formal and informal social controls. Individuals internalise a moral sense as they develop through childhood and adolescence. It is acquired through a secure attachment to their families and to the surrounding culture, through which they learn the elementary codes of human behaviour and the relation between acts and their consequences. But in recent years there has been a comprehensive breakdown of such attachments. Family life has become conditional and contingent; employment is either insecure or non-existent; religious belief has been eroded; schools, both in what they teach and the way they teach it, increasingly abandon children to their own devices.
>
> Instead of authority, firm rules and fixed boundaries which define the world as something intelligible to which the child can become attached, there is now merely an endlessly shifting landscape of subjectivity and ambiguity. The child has become an autonomous and solitary individual, left alone to construct his or her own meaning from the world …
>
> There has been a breakdown in moral transmission from one generation to the next. In the adult world, both parents and their surrogates – teachers, social workers and increasingly the judiciary and other members of the establishment – are retreating from the parental role of promoting the care, control and development of children. In particular, they display a failure to recognise the need for clear moral judgments, discipline and punishment as part of a child's social learning process. Their retreat from this agenda marks a retreat from the principal duty of adults to socialise a child.
>
> (Phillips, 1996, pp.270–1)

Phillips argues for a greater use of discipline towards young (and potential) offenders, including punishments for misdeeds. She sees this is as 'an essential constituent of parental love', since offenders in the late twentieth century were crying out for discipline and for proper parenting, but instead all they received was 'indifference masquerading as benevolence' (1996, p.280). Seen in this light, punishment is 'the act not of a harsh but of a caring society' in that it presupposes that the offender is attached to values defining 'his' identity as a moral being (1996, p.281). Once again, we see an emphasis on the central role of healthy, disciplined, 'natural' families in overcoming what Phillips terms 'the culture of individualism' and the associated moral crisis, and in promoting a cohesive society.

Green on welfare and community beyond the welfare state

In *Community Without Politics* David Green (1996) offered what he terms a New Right market perspective on welfare and community. Here we focus on three aspects of his analysis: the critique of the welfare state; the appeal to a common morality; and the rediscovery of the forgotten UK tradition of civic associatism.

The critique of the welfare state

Green argues that the past hundred years in the UK have taught us the crucial lesson that the purpose of government is not the management of people's lives, such as was tried by the Beveridgean welfare state, but rather the creation of conditions for self-management in mutual but voluntary co-operation with others. 'Experience this century has surely taught us that political caring is a poor substitute for the mutual caring of civil society, and political solidarity an inadequate replacement for the sense of belonging that derives from the acceptance of a moral tradition to which all subscribe, rich and poor alike' (Green, 1996, pp.vii–viii).

In line with much New Right thinking (see **Lewis, 1998b**), Green sees the welfare state as the enemy of freedom and the creator of dependency. However, Green wishes to argue that atomized individualism alone is not the answer, since the free society rests not just on liberty but also on the acceptance of duty to the community.

The appeal to a common morality

Green questions the notion that a concern with morals is necessarily authoritarian and, in line with communitarian philosophers such as MacIntyre, argues for acting morally 'out of habit':

> If the moral system most appropriate to a free society is habitual, then the importance of the family and other intermediate associations becomes easier to see. An habitual morality is essentially a practical way of living which is learnt or acquired by coping or emulating others ... Above all, such a moral system is the possession of people, that is of civil society. It stands or falls by the efforts of each person going about his daily life, upholding or not upholding the virtues it embodies. Everyone counts. And this is its relevance for liberty. Because such a moral system rests on daily face-to-face practice, it is less prone to manipulation by the authorities.
>
> (Green, 1996, pp.26–7)

The rediscovery of the forgotten UK tradition of civic associatism

Green (1996, p.130) goes on to draw lessons from the past, from 'our shared tradition' in the UK before the welfare state. In particular he celebrates the philanthropic ethos of the Victorian period in which there was 'community without politics', which is defined as 'a sense of obligation to help each other without degrading the recipient' and a sense of duty without rights. (For a different interpretation see **Mooney, 1998**.) Green concludes that the past offers a model for a brighter future for the UK, namely a welfare community without the welfare state.

Read Extract 2.2, which is taken from Green's *Community Without Politics*. As you read, consider the following questions:

1 According to Green, what was the nature of the 'forgotten tradition' in pre-welfare state UK society, and how long did it last?

2 What was the balance between rights and duties for those receiving support from the parish?

3 What alternatives to public assistance emerged in this tradition?

4 What are the lessons of the past for future public policy on welfare?

Extract 2.2 Green: 'Community without politics'

The ethos of community without politics

The ethos which prevailed before the welfare state, may be summarised as follows. From medieval times it was accepted that the state (in the form of the parish authorities) had an obligation to prevent starvation. It is common to date the poor law from the Elizabethan legislation of 1601, but as the Royal Commission on the Poor Laws of 1909 found, the obligation to assist the poor has common-law origins pre-dating the Norman Conquest. By the early fourteenth century, 200 years before the earliest Tudor legislation, the tradition of parish relief was well established ... It was possible for a parish officer who allowed an individual to starve in his locality to be prosecuted for manslaughter. It is significant that this requirement was a *duty* placed on the poor law authorities. A duty naturally implies a *right* to assistance, but it had a different effect from a modern *welfare right*, not least because conditions were always attached to receipt of support. In particular, the able-bodied were always expected to perform some work.

Above all, it was also considered something of a disgrace to resort to the parish, and consequently private philanthropy took responsibility for protecting people from having to turn to the poor law. In addition, there were many whose low income put them in danger of having to rely on either the poor law or charity, who took steps to avoid both. They formed mutual aid associations to allow them to create a shared fund on which they could draw in hard times.

Could this model serve as a basis for modern reform? It is obviously utopian in the short run. But I believe it is the ideal to keep in mind as we confront the manifest failings of state welfare.

Public policy should seek to foster a renewal of this three-part ethos of organised welfare: (1) a certain safety net as the minimum, maintained by government; (2) above the safety net a public but not political domain achieved by people assuming responsibility for their less fortunate fellows in a spirit of mutual respect; and (3) a tradition of mutual aid for those who intended to avoid resort not only to the state but also to charity. All this was in addition to the informal assistance of family, neighbours and friends, not to mention commercial insurance.

(Green, 1996, pp.133–4)

For Green the 'forgotten tradition' of the ethos of 'community without politics' stretched a long way back into UK (for which read 'English'?) history, to before the Norman Conquest. In particular, this welfare tradition combined both a public and, most important, a private obligation to help those genuinely deserving of help. At the same time there was some stigma to receiving public welfare, and many poor people developed alternative communal, self-help, mutual aid associations to protect themselves during hard times. The balance between rights and duties for those receiving public support in this 'virtuous' past was one in which stringent conditions were attached to receiving support, not least the duty of the able-bodied to work. Green argues that there are clear lessons from the past for a future public policy agenda on welfare. He accepts that there should be a minimal state-maintained safety-net for 'deserving' welfare claimants; however, he argues that a civic culture of philanthropy and mutual aid should be fostered to replace the welfare state.

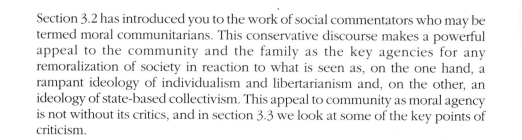

Section 3.2 has introduced you to the work of social commentators who may be termed moral communitarians. This conservative discourse makes a powerful appeal to the community and the family as the key agencies for any remoralization of society in reaction to what is seen as, on the one hand, a rampant ideology of individualism and libertarianism and, on the other, an ideology of state-based collectivism. This appeal to community as moral agency is not without its critics, and in section 3.3 we look at some of the key points of criticism.

3.3   Critique of the moral communitarian discourse

You should now re-read the notes you have made on the moral communitarian discourse of Etzioni, Dennis, Phillips and Green (see Activity 2.3) and consider:

1   What are their shared themes and concerns?

2   What common points of criticism might you make of their moral communitarian discourse on community and welfare?

We would highlight the following main points of both commonality and criticism of the moral communitarian arguments on community and welfare. You may well have noted points that we have failed to address.

The discourse of moral communitarianism may be characterized as being morally authoritarian because of the following assumptions and limitations:

■   A critique of personal rights and a call for duties.

■   A political and moral rallying call for a return to 'the traditional family' as the basis for social welfare.

■   An emphasis on one moral community as the representation of the national popular at the expense of a recognition of the volatility, plurality and diversity of identities in the late twentieth century and beyond.

- A desire to return to a traditional and nostalgic rose-tinted past.

- The neglect of power structures in human societies, or at least a naturalization of hierarchically ordered social relations (particularly in the family).

- The glorification of past solidaristic communities, together with a failure to conceptualize the crucial importance of struggles against oppression in the creation of collectivist, but also exclusivist, communities, such as the traditional working-class communities.

- A moral solution offered for the ills of society (involving an injunction to rebuild society from the moral dimension), to the neglect of an analysis of the material conditions of existence.

■ ■ ■

Within the popular and moralizing communitarian discourse there is a vision of a unitary, homogeneous community sustained by strongly held moral certainties. This vision celebrates mono-culturalism and the setting of a morally prescriptive agenda for the social exclusion of marginalized and 'deviant' categories of people. At the core of this discourse is a particular vision based on an *essentialist* view of human nature (**Clarke and Cochrane, 1998**), in which there is a conservative fear of disorderliness. Community as an orchestrating principle of welfare appears to act through the naturalized practices of familial self-help groups, philanthropy and voluntarism, supported when necessary by the enabling or enforcing state. Campbell (1995, p.51) appears to capture moral communitarianism's particular representation of the reformed 'public' when she argues that: 'Communitarianism celebrates a holy trinity of family, community and nation, as if community represented a halcyon pasture, small but perfectly formed, an immaculately conceived domain of homogeneous kinships, shared interests and common histories.'

3.4 Beyond community: radical left pluralism and the struggle for inclusive communities

This section focuses on the moral and political discourse of commentators who may be grouped together as radical left pluralists. Radical left pluralism attempts to move beyond the idea of *community* in the singular and exclusive sense to focus on the struggle for *communities* in radically plural and inclusive senses. First we examine the radical critique of conservative authoritarianism in general, and of moral communitarianism in particular, articulated by Stuart Hall and Bea Campbell. We then focus on the centrality of the struggles against oppression in the politics of community and welfare in the work of Jeffrey Weeks and Ray Pahl. We conclude by offering a critique of the radical left pluralist discourse on communities and welfare.

Section 2 made it clear that there is no consensus as to what constitutes a community. And just as there is no consensus over the definition of the concept of community, the figure of the community does not belong to any specific ideological position or political persuasion.

Radical left pluralism is critical of discourses of conservative authoritarianism (such as moral communitarianism), arguing instead for a political and welfare strategy of social inclusion based on the struggles of diverse communities and

radical left
pluralism

inclusion

87

the democratic, self-governing associations of civil society. McLennan (1995, p.91) described civil society as: 'that complex realm of social intercourse, social formation and moral-political action which is theorized as being both ungoverned by the formal institutions of the state and irreducible to the logic of the dominant mode of production.' The term 'radical' implies criticism of traditional ways of thinking and acting: the opposite of conservative. In this context we are dealing with a radicalism of the Left rather than of the Right (such as Thatcherism). 'Pluralism' in this context implies the recognition of the importance of differences and diversity, that modern societies are made up of many different groups, households and communities. The main thrust of radical left pluralism is the struggle to valorize *communities* rather than the celebration of *the* community. We might therefore say that this discourse represents the attempt to pluralize the debate on community. Some radical left pluralists understand community as always in a process of formation, as part of the attempt to forge (new) political constituencies. The radical discourse on community politics on which we now focus may be best seen as an articulating practice (in the sense of having the ability to express oneself fluently and coherently), and therein lie both its strengths and its weaknesses.

ACTIVITY 2.8

The rest of section 3.4 contains outlines of the arguments presented by four proponents of radical left pluralism: Stuart Hall, Bea Campbell, Ray Pahl and Jeffrey Weeks. As in Activity 2.3, you should note the main arguments and your own criticisms of the positions presented. You will use these notes in Activity 2.12.

You may find it helpful to use a grid such as this for your notes.

	Main arguments	Critique of arguments
Hall		
Campbell		
Pahl		
Weeks		

3.4.1 Struggles for communal reciprocity and the critique of moral authoritarianism

The moral communitarian discourse discussed in section 3.2 met with some harsh criticism from radical commentators such as Stuart Hall (1993) and Bea Campbell (1993). For some, the logic of its argument leads to the regimentation of opinion, the repression of dissent and the institutionalization of intolerance, all in the name of morality.

You should now read Extract 2.3 by Stuart Hall. In this extract Hall is responding to an early 1990s' policy initiative of the then Prime Minister, John Major, known as 'back to basics'. 'Back to basics' may be viewed as a populist conservative appeal to the notion of one community and one moral order. In reading the extract, consider the following questions:

1   What does Hall identify as the major weaknesses in the Right's 'back to basics' programme of the early 1990s?

2   What does Hall see as the alternative progressive vision of how people might live together?

Extract 2.3 Hall: 'Basic instinct off target'

John Major reaches for the popular Thatcherite, commonsense themes of crime, law and order, family breakdown, and social disintegration, which he calls Back to Basics. In this sense he attempts to combine the impossible – respectability and enterprise. By saying combine these, I refer to the people who thought that, by driving enterprise far enough, it would completely undermine any sense of tradition; of an organic belongingness to society; of the fabric of society; and to some extent that has happened. It is therefore the right who are responsible for the breakdown of the fabric of UK society, and not the left, or 1960s permissiveness.

This makes it more difficult to identify what has happened to the social fabric. It has to do with resources, with the disadvantaged groups, and different constituencies in society. But it also has to do with the breakdown of the reciprocity between individuals, with the diminution of the possibility of evoking any responsibility that we might have for one another. There is only one political and moral force that has been in business over the past 14 years, which has eaten away at the cement of social reciprocity, and that is the Thatcherite project.

That is not just 'big C' Conservatism, nor even an old conservatism – old conservatives know what reciprocity is. For them it is when people tug their forelocks – an attitude that doesn't belong in the 20th century – but if you say reciprocity to the hard-faced men who are at the leading edge of restoring the Thatcherite project, they don't know what you are talking about. They don't know how to cost it, or how to raise funds for it, or where to find it.

The concept has been eroded as the result of a systematic set of practices and ideologies. I have been accused of exaggerating the ideological thrust of Thatcherism. That is because the left has never really understood that ideologies are ideas which organise people's behaviour and conduct.

It is generally difficult to make any distinction between the philosophies through which people understand the world, and the practices through which they operate in it. And, in Britain, we have been engaged in practices, discourses and ideologies that have systematically downgraded the concept of the social and the reciprocity between individuals and groups, which constitute society.

We have thought a good deal about getting rid of what seems to have held us back, but we have not yet thought about how we can construct a new set of relationships. Consider the position of voluntary organisations and political parties. Voluntary organisations, many of which are into extremely important social questions but don't have the same kind of political representative function as political parties, have mainly increased their support and membership over the last decade, while the formal political parties have declined.

It cannot be said, therefore, that this society does not involve itself, want to play an active part in issues which touch the public realm, or is not a joining society. The nature of membership may have changed, but it is a society which gives enormously to charity, for example. Therefore the notion of coming into the public realm in a way which attaches people to an organisation, and begins to open that dialogue between the represented and those who represent, can still be structured in the modern political world.

This is the critical relationship of political representation, without which the function of political parties will inevitably decline. Like the nation state, political parties don't disappear, they just lumber around the stage, able to do less and less, a kind of encumbrance, like giant dinosaurs.

The urgent need now is to find the political forms in which the different projects are stitched together into something which looks like an alternative to the whole way of life that Thatcherism has been offering us and failing to establish.

Only a profound and deep vision, which has a political programme and economic rationale, but is also able to provide alternative models for how people live with one another, will do. It must also address how we deal with difference, and how we constitute relationships amongst ourselves.

Only this will provide a sufficiently powerful countervailing alternative to the historical base on which the Back to Basics populism of Major and the Tories is founded ...

(Hall, 1993, p.24)

COMMENT

Hall argues that the main weakness of the Conservative government's 'back to basics' agenda of 1993 is that it ignores the consequences of its own Thatcherite project: the decline in reciprocity and social solidarity. The 'back to basics' agenda also ignores the crucial social context of the rise in crime, particularly the breakdown of communal networks of support for the most vulnerable sections of working-class youth. Hall offers an alternative 'progressive' vision of how people might live together. In particular, Hall's radical left pluralist discourse suggests that people need to be released from the bonds of traditionalist thinking and develop responsibilities in open and free ways as 'democratic citizens'. He also argues for a reaffirmation of reciprocity between groups and individuals, and that the bonds of reciprocity be developed through voluntary actions and associations. Finally, Hall makes the case for a new politics based on open dialogue between representatives and the represented. In Hall's (1993) words: 'The left has to show how adults can release themselves from the bonds of traditionalist forms of living and thinking, and still be responsible for others in a free and open way. It needs a notion of democratic citizenship.'

■ ■ ■

Campbell on the decline of working-class communities and the 'gender war' in the late twentieth-century UK

Bea Campbell (1993) offered a feminist analysis of the disorders of 1991 which occurred in a number of working-class communities. She argues that most writers on community ignore the significance of the gendered fissures between men and women, not least in the once working-class communities. Campbell

(1993, p.202) states that unemployment has revealed 'a mode of masculinity whereas the common-sense notion has been that it causes a crisis of masculinity … Difference is reasserted in a refusal to co-operate in the creation of a democratic domesticity.' In apparent alliance with the anti-feminist Dennis discussed in section 3.2, Campbell highlights the selfish and aggressive irresponsibility – expressed in a cult of machismo and brute force – of young males in many of the UK's deprived housing estates. That said, unlike Dennis, Campbell prioritizes material factors such as unemployment, poverty and political marginalization, as well as internecine harassment, in producing these brutish 'lads'. Gender is to the fore in Campbell's (1993, p.244) condemnation of the lads and her celebration of the communal struggles of women: 'They [the lads] could penetrate anything while they themselves remained impregnable. What they admired and serviced was the criminalized brotherhood; what they harassed and hurt was community politics. It was an entirely and explicitly gendered formation.' In contrast: 'The redoubts of active citizenship on these estates were run by women whose improvized self-help systems denied their reputation as lairs inhabited by an inert underclass' (Campbell, 1993, p.247).

The possibility of community, and a progressive welfare strategy in the UK's most deprived and criminalized estates, thus rests in the hands of women. 'Solidarity and self-help are sustained by networks that are … open, expansive, egalitarian and incipiently democratic. Their challenge is to the systems that bear upon their local life. Crime and coercion are sustained by men. Solidarity and self-help are sustained by women. It is as stark as that' (Campbell, 1993, p.319).

This is an explicitly gendered account of communal conflict and resistance. It is also an important analysis because it raises issues about the links between, first, how processes of democratization might deal with social difference and, second, how it might do so without denying tensions and inequalities in real communities. It certainly does not underestimate the problem of democratic, inclusive community building.

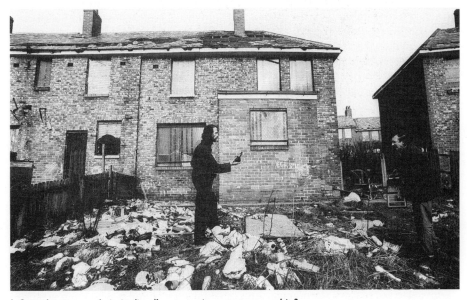

Informal economy: 'criminalized' community entrepreneurship?

3.4.2 Towards a new politics of community: the work of Pahl and Weeks

Both Ray Pahl and Jeffrey Weeks try to offer a vision of communities in late modern societies that moves beyond what they see as the romanticized and regressive appeals of moral communitarians such as Etzioni and Dennis (see section 3.2). Pahl finds Etzioni's philosophy 'sociologically unconvincing', since it ignores the material conditions of existence of communities and avoids any analysis of power and conflict and of divisiveness in communities. Pahl (1995, p.21) argues that the sense of community in the singular is now historically redundant, and he promotes what he terms the 'friendly society': 'Community in the past was imposed on people, being largely based on involuntary relationships. Now people *choose* their associates – and perhaps more importantly, choose with whom not to associate.'

ACTIVITY 2.10

Pahl's alternative approach to Etzioni's philosophy is developed in Extract 2.4, which was written before the election of a Labour government in 1997. In reading this extract, you should consider the following questions:

1 What does Pahl mean by the importance of the distinction between what deprived and oppressed minorities actually do as against what they ought to do?

2 Pahl questions the idea of seeing the (patriarchal) family as the only source of social welfare, cohesion and control. What other supportive bonds does Pahl highlight?

3 What distinction does Pahl draw between individualism and individuality?

Extract 2.4 Pahl: 'Friendly society'

If the communitarian philosophy fails to be sociologically convincing, what is to be put in its place? My own inclination is to start with what is, rather than what *ought* to be. If the desire is to celebrate and support those who engage in communal and collective endeavours then we should see who *actually* does this, rather than those who *ought* to do it. In practice those who are most in need of supportive and communal activity are lone parents. Those in the very category pilloried by communitarians are setting up support groups for themselves, and various other cooperative activities for others in the same place. As Carol Stack has shown in *All our Kin*, lone, black mothers in a deprived urban environment in the US can create valuable and essential solidarities. The same can be shown for many deprived and oppressed minorities.

Such minorities may express their solidarity in opposition to the majority and, as long as they remain conscious of their excluded status, the sense of identity will remain. New forms of exclusion create new potentials for identity. These new solidarities of the oppressed are likely to be in inner city areas – often the very areas that cause communitarians the most dismay.

Those who are most praised by communitarians – the doting, caring parents taking their childcare very responsibly, and devoting considerable time to their children, have little time for much else. Both partners are likely to be in employment – even if only on a part-time basis for the woman. They probably have to spend much of their week in tiring travel, commuting to work, collecting children, visiting relatives, driving to out of town shopping centres or taking their children swimming or ice-skating. At evenings or weekends they are more likely to be more exhausted than active citizens. The harassed, time-challenged middle mass are obliged to be highly selective in how they choose their friends and associates.

Those who do have the time, energy and inclination to engage in public-spirited work are more likely to be single. The divorcees and the lone parents are more likely to be younger: the widows, widowers and pensioners will be older. Some vigorous widows in their 60s and 70s can make fine community activists if not over-committed as grandmothers.

One of the massive fallacies of the current debate is that because of the decline of 'the traditional community' social and geographical mobility has made social atoms of us all. Politicians and pundits frequently fall into the trap of seeing the family as the only putative source of social cohesion and control, so higher rates of divorce and the rapid growth of lone-parent families is seen as a dangerous dilution of social glue. The answer by the communitarians and the father-fans, like Norman Dennis and A H Halsey, writing for the Institute of Economic Affairs, is to seek to strengthen the male breadwinner role for the sake of his dependents. Yet surely there can be no return to the patriarchal working-class family: all the survey material on the younger generation supports this, as Helen Wilkinson's Demos pamphlet *No Turning Back* recently showed.

This obsession with the ideological connotations surrounding community and family has led to one of the most powerful supportive bonds of modern society being neglected. The reason most of us are not mere social atoms fighting our corner in competitive market is that we have our friends, our mates, our support group. Girlfriends and boyfriends come and go; children grow up and find their own identities elsewhere, partners come and partners go, but friends provide the social glue. Sometimes, it is true, siblings or cousins can be friends. But, more often, best friends comfort in time of bereavement or the break-up of a relationship. We need our friends and our friends need us. The idea that fraternity is limited to male bonded trade unionists is a sexist anachronism …

Politicians have probably neglected to consider friendship seriously because they cannot see clearly how to fit friends into an institutional context. Family-supportive policies are one thing … but friend-friendly policies – what on earth would that entail? Sociologists have tended to abstract from relationships and have studied types of social networks and the forms and norms of reciprocity. Such language does not resonate with politicians who may be prepared to learn economists' jargon, but see no point in doing the same for anthropology or sociology. However, if politicians recognised the social importance of friendship it would do much to avoid the alienating consequences of much political rhetoric.

Fearful of overtones of Thatcherite individualism based on competition and greed, Tony Blair wants to substitute social-ism for a selfish and uncaring individualism. In doing this he is likely to make a very dangerous blunder by misunderstanding how people are actually behaving in their everyday lives. They are being social as individuals. Their individuality is vitally important to them. This distinction between individualism and individuality is crucial, and is the vital missing element of discussion in contemporary politics. Misguidedly, Tony Blair has latched on to community and communitarianism as alternatives to the discarded individualist ideology of the 1980s. The danger is that he will miss the significance of individuality and so people may fear that their own individuality may not be so easily nourished and developed under his social-ism.

Individuality implies diversity, tolerance and creativity. We flourish with our friends. I suggest that Tony Blair should articulate how he would develop a more user-friendly style of government that would encourage more diversity and spontaneity.

Instead of a rather pious couple-ism and familism, the Labour Party should lead and reflect the mood of the 1990s – people are not social atoms anonymously colliding in a harsh and competitive environment. They are generally warm and friendly people trying to come to terms with themselves and their relationships. They need support, not censure. There is no need to fall for a phoney communitarianism: what is needed is an acceptance that most people are struggling on as best they can with the help of their friends.

There was something in Thatcherism that did appeal to the individualism of the British but it became badly infected with manic ideological overtones. It would be a pity if, in reaction to this, there were a similar uncritical commitment to an alternative unproductive ideology. Don't see divorce statistics and the growth of lone-parent households as indicators of the lack of social cohesion. Rather see how friendships and the solidarity of single mothers are creating new, better and more equal bonds in society.

The mood of the late 1990s is surely that people are engaged in a struggle to find an identity for themselves which is sensitive to them as they really are. They reject the notion that they should subordinate themselves to collective categories. As we know from our own personal experience, our attachment to collectives is mediated by our *personal* experience. It is an obvious, yet crucial, insight that people read collectivities through their experience as individuals. Simply because people may use collective forms to assert their identities, it would be a great mistake to assume that this implies uniformities of identity. By being wary of the selfish self of the 1980s, we are in danger of ignoring the *self-conscious self* of the 1990s.

Despite many in the Labour Party seeing the dangers of this ideological individualism, it is tragic that so few have recognised the deep-seated urge for individuality among people in our society. There is still time to make amends. Let us move beyond communitarianism to a diverse, tolerant and friendly society based on creative individuality.

(Pahl, 1995, pp.21–2)

COMMENT

Pahl argues that deprived and oppressed minorities such as lone parents are expressing solidarity through, for example, self-help support groups, often in opposition to the 'moral majority'. Thus new forms of exclusion, or at best conditional inclusions, create the potential for new forms of identity and belonging as welfare subjects (see **Lewis, 1998b**). Pahl also contends that the obsession with the (patriarchal) family has led to the neglect of sources of cohesion and control associated with the bonds of friendship. Finally, according to Pahl, individualism is chiefly based on greed and competition. It is, in other words, an ideology of selfishness. Individuality, on the other hand, implies diversity, tolerance and creativity. It is arguably most manifest in our relationships with friends (as against the dominant welfare policy discourse of 'coupleism' and 'familism'). Pahl concludes that we should not attempt to subordinate the individual to any uniform identity.

■ ■ ■

Jeffrey Weeks (1996) has also made an important contribution to radical left pluralist thinking. While he focuses on the emergence of a new politics and sense of community among gay and lesbian people in the post-AIDS decades of the late twentieth century, his arguments have a wider relevance.

You should now read Extract 2.5, which is taken from a paper which Weeks entitled 'The idea of a sexual community'. As you read, consider the following questions:

1   What does Weeks see as the major appeal of communitarianism and community for people in the late twentieth century?

2   What is meant by the term 'critical community', and what are its main features compared to 'given' or traditional communities?

3   What does Weeks mean by community being 'a necessary fiction'?

4   How might his argument be applied to other oppressed groups or communities, such as disabled people or people from ethnic minorities?

Extract 2.5 Weeks: 'The idea of a sexual community'

[Community] attempts both to express social realities and to offer an aspiration towards something better, more inclusive and tangible. In the form of contemporary communitarianism, the pursuit of community suggests a revulsion against the coldness and impersonality, the instrumentality and narrow self interest, of abstract individualism with its associated marketisation and commodification of human bonds. The idea of community, in contrast to social atomisation, suggests that men and women should be members and not strangers, should have ties and belongings that transcend the monad [or individual unit] …

The challenge for modern advocates of community, therefore, is to imagine community without either neo-tribalism or self immolation. The key issue, I would argue, is not whether community, but what sort of community, and what sort of identity, are appropriate at any particular time. Michel Foucault distinguishes between three concepts of community: a *given community*, a *tacit community* and a *critical community*.

> a given community arises from an identification: 'I am an X'. Tacit community is the materially-rooted system of thought that makes X a possible object of identification; and critical community sees this system of thought as singular or contingent, finds something 'intolerable' about it, and starts to refuse to participate in it. [Foucault cited in Rajchman, 1991]

In the contemporary world, 'given' – or traditional – communities are losing their moral density as old values crumble and uncertainty rules … A critical community, on the other hand, results from a problematisation of a given or latent identity. It is open to new experiences and ways of being, which make new subjectivities possible. At its best, I shall argue, the idea of a sexual community as it is evoked in contemporary radical sexual political discourse embraces this notion of a critical community.

In other words, it is because homosexuality is not the norm, is stigmatised, that a sense of community transcending specific differences, has emerged. It exists because participants in it feel it does and should exist. It is not geographically fixed. It is criss-crossed by many divisions. But a sort of diasporic consciousness does exist because people believe it exists. And this belief has material and cultural effects …

Politically, radical sexual communities and their associated movements point in two different directions at once – or at least embrace two distinct political moments: what I call the 'moment of transgression', and the 'moment of citizenship'. The 'moment of transgression' is the moment of challenge to the traditional or received order of sexual life: the assertion of different identities, different life-styles, and the building of oppositional communities. In its recent form it has given rise to 'queer politics', which has sought to break with what has been perceived as the caution of contemporary gay politics with its integrationist approaches. The 'moment of citizenship' is precisely this movement towards inclusion, towards redefining the polity to incorporate fully those who have felt excluded. Its characteristic emphasis has been on the claiming of civil rights, formal equality – and most recently, in continental Europe at least, on the demand for 'partnership rights' for same sex couples. On the surface at least they seem radically different strategies, and find expression in different organisational forms: for example, in the UK, in the differences between the confrontationalist politics of Outrage! and the lobbying approach of Stonewall …

I have argued elsewhere that the idea of a sexual identity is a fiction (because it is based on the cultural construction of plausible narratives to make sense of individual lives). But it is a necessary fiction because it offers the possibility of social agency in a context where equal access to social goods is denied. In the same way, the idea of a sexual community may be a fiction, but it is a necessary fiction: an imagined community, an invented tradition which enables and empowers. It provides the context for the articulation of identity, the vocabulary of values through which ways of life can be developed, the accumulated skills by which new possibilities can be explored and hazards negotiated, and the context for the emergence of social movements and political campaigns which seek to challenge the existing order.

There are, of course, dangers. The new elective communities can be as exclusive and stifling as traditional ones. Social pluralism and a proliferation of communities do not necessarily guarantee variety or autonomy for all members. The co-existence of different communities depends upon a recognition that the condition of toleration of one's own way of life is a recognition of the validity of other ways of life. That, in turn, requires that communities guarantee a freedom of exit and of voice for their members. The communities built around sexuality are no less likely than others to develop their own norms which may exclude as well as include.

But having said that, it should also be acknowledged that in the contemporary world, with its deep sense of uncertainty around values, the idea of a sexual community has developed because of a conviction that it is only through the enhancement of a collective identity that individual autonomy can be realised.

That is not all that could be said about the idea of community in general, or about sexual communities in particular. But it is enough, I hope, to illustrate my main point: in the contemporary world, the idea of a sexual community is both a necessary and an inevitable one. We cannot do without it.

Reference

Rajchman, J. (1991) *Truth and Eros: Foucault, Lacan and the Question of Ethics*, London and New York, Routledge.

(Weeks, 1996, pp.71–4, 78, 82–4)

COMMENT

Weeks explores the many and complex meanings of community through the perspective of gay and lesbian people and their struggles against oppression, discrimination and stigma. According to Weeks, the idea of community has a particularly strong appeal to people in the late twentieth century; it offers an antidote to the impersonality of much modern life and a means of collective belonging – and welfare support – beyond that of individualism or the state. Weeks argues that the notion of a 'critical community' is important in problematizing a given or latent identity associated with 'traditional' communities. The idea of a critical community also opens up new possibilities for belonging as subjects, particularly for members of oppressed groups, in their struggles against exclusion.

Weeks concludes that the idea of community is 'a necessary fiction', since it opens up the possibility of social agency where equal access to social goods, such as the provision of adequate welfare rights, is denied. For example, the idea of the gay and lesbian community may enable and empower individuals in a way that both enhances collective identity and individual autonomy. In Weeks, as well as in other writers on oppressed communities (see Gilroy, 1997), we can see an emphasis in the radical left pluralist discourse on plural communities of people not rooted in a specific locality or geographical area or fixed culture. This is in contrast to the discourse of moral communitarianism and suggests a radical reworking of traditional notions of 'the public'. Furthermore, the challenge of such a discourse for the future organization, provision and delivery of social welfare would seem immense.

■ ■ ■

3.5   Critique of the radical left pluralist discourse on communities

ACTIVITY 2.12

You should now re-read the notes you have made on the radical left pluralist writings of Hall, Campbell, Pahl and Weeks (see Activity 2.8) and then consider the following questions:

1   What common arguments are presented by these authors?
2   What common points of criticism would you make of their radical left pluralist discourse on community and welfare?

COMMENT

We would suggest the following main points of criticism of the radical left pluralist arguments on community and welfare. You may well have noted points that we have failed to address.

The radical left pluralist discourse on community and welfare may be criticized on the basis of the following shared assumptions and limitations:

■   It may be viewed as utopian and unrealistic given the inherent conflicts and sources of exclusion in modern societies.

■   It would seem to have a vision of a nation of communities, and there is the problem of how such a society could be held together without some overarching, unifying norms.

■   It may underestimate the growth of individualism in modern societies.

■   It may fail to address the problem of the power of big institutions and organizations over the struggles of oppressed minorities.

■   It may not take account of restricted rights to membership of a welfare community in the context of globalizing conditions.

■   It may underestimate the capacity for 'elective' communities to be oppressive.

In summary, whereas the moral communitarian discourse is held together by a conservative and essentialist view of human nature, this second vision arguably has a constructionist view of human beings. Accordingly, in the radical left pluralist vision of people as members of communities nothing is fixed by nature or tradition. Furthermore, this radical discourse sees the process of forging imagined communities as both a source of activism and a source of (welfare) demands on the state (as opposed to the celebration of voluntarism and self-help in the moral communitarian discourse). Illustrative of such tendencies would be the demands for adequate health and social care and rights for HIV-positive people from the gay community. There is, then, an implicit notion of the public realm as something that has demands made upon it.

■ ■ ■

4   Conclusion

This chapter has not explored in depth particular social policies that have embraced or targeted community. However, in section 2 we referred to a number of policies, developed since the 1960s in particular, which deploy community in a myriad of different ways. Section 3 considered some of the ways in which community has been used in the 1990s as part of competing attempts to rethink the relationship between social groups and the state. We suggested that community has become a key element in new political languages that seek to dominate ways of thinking about society and social arrangements.

Community has long been socially constructed and represented as central to social life, as a key element in the national popular. We would suggest that this process will continue, albeit in ways which attempt to reimagine community in a non-place bounded sense, and which recognize the multiplicity and diversity of communities.

Community remains highly seductive as a means of promoting social justice and regulation. Punishment in the community, or care in the community, despite the problems which plague such ideas, serve to both legitimate certain strategies and cast them in a positive (community) light. Community, along with the consumer and the citizen, will continue to be socially constructed as popular ways of imagining social relations.

This chapter has shown that community tends to be deployed along with other socially constructed figures, notably the family and nation. Taken together, family, community and nation – an unholy trinity of contested and problematized notions – serve to structure ways of thinking about 'the social' or 'the public'. In the government of Tony Blair elected in 1997, the language of community, family and nation have been ever present. The Labour government's discourse is one which continually stresses personal responsibilities, albeit in ways which borrow from the language of the New Right. Building communities founded upon the obligations of responsible families has become central to Labour's strategy to 'modernize' UK society. For Blair, 'the search is on to reinvent community for a modern age, true to core values of fairness, co-operation and responsibility' (*The Guardian*, 29 January 1996). Community becomes a key channel through which government will be enacted. Social justice is reworked as community and individual obligation.

The different positions on community considered in section 3 are part of a struggle for a new moral economy, how 'the public' might be imagined in relation to social and welfare policies, and over the role of the state. This struggle is ongoing and volatile. The competing perspectives construct very different senses of 'the public' and 'the social'. In conservative moral communitarianism, communities are naturalized as pre-social units within which welfare needs are identified and met. In the radical left pluralist variant, community is used to make political claims against the state, and demands for public provision. Despite these differences, both discourses share an abandonment of the universalist principles of the Beveridgean welfare state and a growing awareness of its inability to meet the needs of many people and groups. In this respect both moral communitarianism and radical left pluralism share an opposition to statist forms of social policy and welfare organization. Here, community is posited as an experience somewhere between the state and the individual. Although the reasons why may be very different, community remains highly seductive across the political spectrum.

Community, in all its competing and divergent senses and interpretations is, above all, socially constructed. This inescapably throws up issues of inclusions and exclusions, and of responsibility and autonomy. We should continue to bear in mind that the new language of community and the communitarian debate in the late twentieth century took place amidst deepening social and economic inequality, in a period when social polarization, in opposition to the rhetoric of 'fairness', 'cohesion' and 'integration', was an ever-increasing feature of UK and other European societies.

Further reading

On the seduction of community as an ideological appeal see Anderson (1983). For a critique of the political uses of community and communitarianism see Frazer and Lacey (1993). Hoggett (1997) offers a valuable collection of essays on the interface between community and policy. On the various meanings of pluralism see McLennan (1995).

References

Anderson, B. (1983) *Imagined Communities*, London, Verso.

Barnes, M. (1997) *Care, Communities and Citizens*, London, Longman.

Barr, A. (1995) 'Empowering communities – beyond fashionable rhetoric? Some reflections on Scottish experience', *Community Development Journal*, vol.30, no.2, pp.121–32.

Beaton, L. (1985) *Shifting Horizons*, London, Canary Press.

Bellos, A. (1997) 'Let our people go-go ... ', *The Guardian*, 15 April, pp.6–7.

Bornat, J. (1993) 'Representations of community', in Bornat, J., Pereira, C., Pilgrim, D. and Williams, F. (eds) *Community Care: A Reader*, London, MacMillan.

Bourke, J. (1994) *Working-class Cultures in Britain, 1860–1960*, London, Routledge.

Bowring, F. (1997) 'Communitarianism and morality: in search of the subject', *New Left Review*, no.222, pp.93–113.

Braithwaite, J. (1989) *Crime, Shame and Re-integration*, Oxford University Press, Oxford.

Brook, E. and Finn, D. (1978) 'Working-class images of society and community studies', in Centre for Contemporary Cultural Studies (eds) *On Ideology*, London, Hutchinson.

Callinicos, A. (1996) 'Betrayal and discontent: Labour under Blair', *International Socialism*, no.72, pp.3–25.

Campbell, B. (1993) *Goliath: Britain's Dangerous Places*, London, Methuen.

Campbell, B. (1995) 'Old fogeys and angry young men', *Soundings,* issue 1, autumn, pp.47–64.

Charles, N. and Davies, C.A. (1997) 'Contested communities: the refuge movement and cultural identities in Wales', *Sociological Review*, vol.45, no.3, pp.416–36.

Christophersen, S. (1994) 'The fortress city', in Amin, A. (ed.) *Post-Fordism: A Reader*, Oxford, Blackwell.

Clarke, J. and Cochrane, A. (1998) 'The social construction of social problems', in Saraga, E. (ed.) *Embodying the Social: Constructions of Difference*, London, Routledge in association with The Open University.

Cochrane, A. (1986) 'Community politics and democracy', in Held, D. and Pollitt, C. (eds) *New Forms of Democracy*, London, Sage.

Cole, I., Gidley, G., Ritchie, C., Simpson, D. and Wishart, B. (1997) *Creating Communities or Welfare Housing?*, Coventry, The Chartered Institute of Housing/ Joseph Rowntree Foundation.

Danziger, N. (1996) *Danziger's Britain*, London, Harper Collins.

Davis, M. (1990) *City of Quartz*, London, Verso.

Dennis, N. (1958) 'The popularity of the neighbourhood community idea', *Sociological Review*, vol.6, no.2, pp.191–206.

Dennis, N. (1993) *Rising Crime and the Dismembered Family*, London, Institute of Economic Affairs.

Dennis, N. (1997) *The Invention of Permanent Poverty*, London, Institute of Economic Affairs.

Dennis, N. and Erdos, G. (1993) *Families Without Fatherhood*, London, Institute of Economic Affairs.

Dennis, N., Henriques, F. and Slaughter, C. (1969) *Coal Is Our Life* (2nd edn), London, Tavistock.

Duffy, K. and Hutchinson, J. (1997) 'Urban policy and the turn to community', *Town Planning Review*, vol.68, no.3, pp.347–62.

Eade, J. (1997) 'Reconstructing places: changing images of locality in Docklands and Spitalfields', in Eade, J. (ed.) *Living the Global City*, London, Routledge.

Etzioni, A. (1994) *The Spirit of Community: The Reinvention of American Society*, New York, Touchstone.

Etzioni, A. (1995) *The Spirit of Community*, London, Fontana.

Frankenberg, R. (1966) *Communities in Britain*, Harmondsworth, Penguin.

Frazer, E. and Lacey, N. (1993) *The Politics of Community*, Hemel Hempstead, Harvester Wheatsheaf.

Gilroy, P. (1987) *There Ain't No Black in the Union Jack*, London, Hutchinson.

Gilroy, P. (1997) 'Diaspora and the detours of identity', in Woodward, K. (ed.) *Identity and Difference*, London, Sage.

Gray, J. (1995) 'Hollowing out the core', *The Guardian*, 8 March, p.26.

Green, D. (1996) *Community Without Politics: A Market Approach to Welfare Reform*, London, Institute of Economic Affairs.

Green, J. and Chapman, A. (1992) 'The British CDP: lessons for today', *Community Development Journal*, vol.27, no.3, pp.242–58.

The Guardian (1995) 'Community spirit', 13 March, 2, pp.10–11.

Hall, S. (1993) 'Basic instinct off target', *The Guardian*, 24 November.

Hill, D.M. (1994) *Citizens and Cities*, Hemel Hempstead, Harvester Wheatsheaf.

Hillery, G.A. (1955) 'Definitions of community: areas of agreement', *Rural Sociology*, vol.20, no.2, pp.111–23.

Hoggett, P. (1997) 'Contested communities', in Hoggett, P. (ed.) *Contested Communities*, Bristol, The Policy Press.

Hughes, G. (1996) 'Communitarianism and law and order', *Critical Social Policy*, vol.16, no.4, pp.17–41.

Hughes, G. (1998) '"Picking over the remains": the welfare state settlements of the post-Second World War UK', in Hughes and Lewis (eds) (1998).

Hughes, G. and Lewis, G. (eds) (1998) *Unsettling Welfare: The Reconstruction of Social Policy*, London, Routledge in association with The Open University.

Johnson, P. (1994) 'Introduction: Britain, 1900–1990', in Johnson, P. (ed.) *20th Century Britain*, London, Longman.

Jordan, B. (1996) *A Theory of Poverty and Social Exclusion*, Cambridge, Polity Press.

Laing, S. (1986) *Representations of Working-Class Life: 1957–1964*, London, MacMillan.

Lansley, S. (1979) *Housing and Public Policy*, London, Croom Helm.

Lasch, C. (1995) *The Revolt of the Elites and the Betrayal of Democracy*, New York, Norton.

Lebeau, V. (1997) 'The worst of all possible worlds?', in Silverstone, R. (ed.) *Visions of Suburbia*, London, Routledge.

Lee, D. and Newby, H. (1983) *The Problem of Sociology*, London, Unwin Hyman.

Lewis, G. (ed.) (1998a) *Forming Nation, Framing Welfare*, London, Routledge in association with The Open University.

Lewis, G. (ed.) (1998b) '"Coming apart at the seams": the crises of the welfare state', in Lewis and Hughes (eds) (1998).

MacIntyre, A. (1981) *After Virtue: A Study of Moral Theory*, London, Duckworth.

McArthur, A. (1995) 'The active involvement of local community residents in strategic community partnerships', *Policy and Politics*, no.23, pp.61–71.

McGrew, A. (1992) 'A global society?', in Hall, S., Held, D. and McGrew, T. (eds) *Modernity and Its Futures*, Cambridge, Polity Press in association with The Open University.

McLennan, G. (1995) *Pluralism*, Buckingham, Open University Press.

McVicar, E. (1990) *One Singer, One Song*, Glasgow, Glasgow City Libraries.

Mooney, G. (1998) '"Remoralizing" the poor?: gender, class and philanthropy in Victorian Britain', in Lewis (ed.) (1998a).

Morris, L. (1998) 'Legitimate membership of the welfare community', in Langan, M. (ed.) *Welfare: Needs, Rights and Risks*, London, Routledge in association with The Open University.

Murray, C. (1990) *Losing Ground*, New York, Arrow.

Murray, C. (1996) 'The underclass', in Muncie, J. and McLaughlin, E. (eds) *Criminological Perspectives*, London, Sage.

Pahl, R. (1995) 'Friendly society', *New Statesman and Society*, 10 March, pp.20–2.

Phillips, M. (1996) *All Must Have Prizes*, London, Little, Brown and Company.

Plant, R. (1978) 'Community: concept, conception and ideology', *Politics and Society*, vol.8, no.1, pp.79–107.

Rawls, J. (1973) *A Theory of Justice*, Oxford, Oxford University Press.

Rose, N. (1996) 'The death of the social? Re-figuring the territory of government', *Economy and Society*, vol.25, no.3, pp.327–56.

Savage, M. and Warde, A. (1993) *Urban Sociology, Capitalism and Modernity*, London, Macmillan.

Scottish Office (1988) *New Life For Urban Scotland*, Edinburgh, HMSO.

Scottish Office (1996) *Partnerships In Regeneration of Urban Scotland*, Edinburgh, HMSO.

Sennett, R. (1996) *The Uses of Disorder*, London, Faber and Faber.

Sharpe, J. (1996) 'Crime, order and historical change', in Muncie, J. and McLaughlin, E. (eds) *The Problem of Crime*, London, Sage.

Smith, J. (1997) 'The ideology of "family and community": New Labour abandons the welfare state', in Panitch, L. (ed.) *The Socialist Register, 1997*, Suffolk, Merlin Press.

Southall Black Sisters (1989) *Against the Grain*, London, Southall Black Sisters.

Stead, J. (1987) *Never the Same Again: Women and the Miners Strike*, London, The Woman's Press.

Steedman, C. (1986) *Landscape for a Good Woman*, London, Virago.

Taylor, I., Evans, I. and Fraser, P. (1996) *A Tale of Two Cities*, London, Routledge.

Tönnies, F. (1957) *Community and Society (1887)*, New York, Harper and Row.

Weeks, J. (1991) 'Pretended family relationships', in Clark, D. (ed.) *Marriage, Domestic Life and Social Change*, London, Routledge.

Weeks, J. (1996) 'The idea of a sexual community', *Soundings*, issue 2, pp.71–84.

Williams, F. (1993) 'Women and community', in Bornat, J., Pereira, C., Pilgrim, D. and Williams, F. (eds) *Community Care: A Reader*, London, Macmillan.

Williams, R. (1988) *Keywords*, Glasgow, Fontana.

Worsley, P. (ed.) (1987) *The New Introducing Sociology*, Harmondsworth, Penguin.

Young, I.M. (1990) 'The ideal of community and the politics of difference', in Nicholson, L. (ed.) *Feminism/Postmodernism*, London, Routledge.

Young, M. and Willmott, P. (1957) *Family and Kinship in East London*, London, Routledge and Kegan Paul.

CHAPTER 3

Citizenship

by Gail Lewis

Contents

1   Introduction

In this chapter we turn our attention to the 'figure' of the citizen and its relation to welfare. As was indicated in the Introduction to this book, 'the citizen' was the pivotal figure in the dominant imagery of the social democratic welfare state. As a result of this it is perhaps inevitable that the idea of citizenship should be central to any discussion of the 'imaginary relations of welfare'. Similarly, the language and imagery of citizenship provided a reference point for arguments both in support of and against the welfare reforms begun in the 1980s. 'Citizenship' has, then, provided a way of constructing competing understandings about the relation between 'the people', the state and welfare services. Given this, there are three main reasons why we are thinking about citizenship in this book:

1   'The citizen' is one way of imagining a link between the state and the individual.

2   Citizenship is a category of belonging which has been central to the construction of boundaries of entitlement and therefore it raises questions about both social *ex*clusions as well as social *in*clusions.

3   Citizenship is a social status which articulates and mediates the entitlements of the individual to state-organized welfare and was the category at the heart of the social democratic welfare state.

In addition to these points, the idea of citizenship – that is, its meaning – became the subject of intense ideological struggle in the late twentieth century. This can be related to a number of factors. First, there were the contestations over, challenges to and demands for full citizenship rights which came from the new social movements. Second, there was the erosion of established entitlements by successive Conservative governments from 1979 onwards and this erosion was accompanied by a radical shift in the 'common sense' about welfare rights. Lastly, there was the challenge to the nation-state – which is the entity to which citizens belong and to which the language of citizenship speaks – by forces of globalization and regional and ethnic 'nationalisms'/'communalisms'.

In this sense, then, discussion of citizenship provides one means through which to explore the socially constructed nature of welfare belongings, entitlements and duties.

1.1   Citizenship and the national popular

Notions and discourses of citizenship are a way of constructing an imagery of forms of social integration within a society. This is so in the dual sense of (i) seeing citizenship status as providing the connective tissue which binds a collection of individuals into a grouping with common interests and promotes harmony among them; and (ii) the formation of a moral community in the sense of the ethical ties binding people together and mediating their rights and obligations. 'Citizenship' as an idea, then, is a means of constructing a 'we' – that is, a group or collectivity bounded by place, status and interest. As such, a connection can be made between citizenship and the idea of the national popular referred to in the Introduction to this book. Let us take a moment to remind

(margin notes: citizenship; moral community; national popular)

ourselves why the Gramscian notion of the national popular (Gramsci, 1971) is seen as relevant to the concerns of this book.

In the Introduction to the book it was stated that the national popular was relevant to our concerns with imagined welfare futures for three main reasons:

1   It alerted us to the various meanings which are attached to 'the nation'.

2   It defined these meanings, understandings and representations of the people and the nation as a legitimate and central arena of *political* struggle.

3   It recognized that social groups construct forms of identification across numerous sets of interests and not just those which are understood to correspond to their economic or ideological *self*-interests.

Seen in this way, the national popular should be understood as both a cultural and a political concept (Forgacs, 1993) and, for the purposes of this chapter, I want to rephrase this to mean that the national popular can be understood to contain three analytically distinct but interrelated elements:

1   It suggests a way of constructing categories of belonging.

2   It suggests the existence of diverse sets of feelings, outlooks and proclivities which attach to analytically discrete social categories within the population.

3   It provides a way of identifying numerous groups, channels and methods of political intervention.

Chapters 1 and 2 have considered what this means for the consideration of the 'consumer' and the 'community' respectively. In this chapter I want to consider how the social, cultural and political figure of the citizen articulates these three **articulate** interrelated elements – by which I mean how both the idea and the discourse of citizenship are deployed to provide a means through which to speak about and connect these elements in an attempt to construct categories of belonging to, constituencies of feeling about, and conduits of political intervention into the field of welfare.

I will consider this process of articulation by organizing the chapter in the following way. In section 2, I offer a brief introduction to the category of citizenship and suggest some of the associations which this term carries. In section 3, I outline the approach put forward by T.H. Marshall in the early 1950s. Marshall's definition of citizenship and his view of its connection to questions of class inequality provided the dominant paradigm framing official and popular understanding about the link between citizenship and social welfare for many decades. In section 4, I look at a recent approach to the promotion of citizenship found in an All Party Parliamentary Commission. For our purposes, the importance of this report lies in the way in which it reflects a shift away from issues of *redistribution*, which were central to Marshall's approach and which characterized the social democratic consensus of the post-1945 welfare state.

Sections 5 and 6 return to two central questions which derive from the Marshallian approach and which are at the heart of competing approaches to citizenship which emerged in the wake of the radical restructuring of social welfare begun in the 1980s. These are, respectively, the link to the question of markets, private initiative and 'the public sphere' (section 5); and the question of gender inequality (section 6). In section 7, the theme of inequality is retained but this time with regard to the tensions which result when citizenship is viewed in relation to the nation-state and in isolation from that nation-state's history. Two issues in particular are considered here. We begin by considering the extent to which British citizenship and nationality up to 1981 could be considered an imperial construction, the effect of which was to organize hierarchically the relative strength of individual nation-states within the Commonwealth. We then go on to consider the potential impact of the European Union (EU) on some of the inequalities which have characterized citizenship in the UK.

Finally, and by way of conclusion, there is a brief consideration of what all this might mean for the imaginary relations of welfare in the UK on the cusp of the twentieth and twenty-first centuries. As you read through the various extracts in the chapter it is important that you recognize their *interpretative* quality. By this I mean that they are examples of how their authors have constructed the *idea* of citizenship and what this status has meant, or might mean, for the provision of and access to welfare services. Moreover, three of the extracts are about particular authors' visions of a *future* system of welfare relations. As such, they exemplify some of the contestations current in the 1990s about how to construct categories of belonging, entitlements to and responsibilities for welfare services and benefits at a time when the conceptions and structures of the social democratic welfare state no longer occupied the position of truth or common sense. The extracts therefore provide a series of illustrations about the imaginary futures of welfare.

2 Citizenship: some introductory remarks

In general terms, the idea of 'citizenship' stretches back to the ancient polities organized around city-states such as those found in Athens and Rome in Classical times – forms of citizenship have therefore existed for many centuries. To say this, however, is not to imply that what is *meant* by citizenship has remained unchanged throughout different epochs and in different states, but before going on to think about some of the characteristics of the liberal conception of citizenship, it is worth noting a number of attributes common to all conceptions of citizenship. Held (1991, pp.20–1) has attempted to delineate such common attributes and suggests the following:

- Citizenship has meant membership of and participation in a bounded entity which is expressed as series of reciprocal rights and duties within that entity.

- As such, citizenship rights are *public* or *social* entitlements which both confer and derive from a social status.

- Despite this social status, these rights are nevertheless conferred upon *individuals*, and this combination constructs an unusual mix of social and individual aspects of political life.

- Citizenship therefore establishes a series of spheres of action which may be legitimately pursued with freedom from interference, constraint or coercion.

These issues direct us towards some important points of tension and conflict to which we will return at various places in the chapter; here I want to continue with a few general remarks. Today perhaps the most common understanding of the meaning of citizenship is that it confers the right to carry a passport issued by a particular nation-state. As citizens, those who hold such passports are both understood as 'belonging' to the issuing country, and afforded the right to travel across the borders of other nation-states. Following from this, we can see that one aspect of citizenship is that it is a legal status defined and conferred by internationally recognized nation-states against which its citizens have entitlements to which they can make claim. In abstract legal terms, all citizens of a state are formally equal and their civil rights (guaranteed by the rule of law) protect their safety and freedom, in the liberal sense of the absence of coercion. A defining distinction between the citizenship associated with such city-states as Athens and Rome and that which characterizes citizenship in the UK today is the ability of all those who hold citizenship status to participate in formal political life through electoral processes: 'Thus participation by citizens in the modern nation-state entails legal membership of a political community based on universal suffrage and therefore also membership of a civil community based on the rule of law' (Barbalet, 1988, p.2).

Defining citizenship in this way clearly reveals its roots in liberalism, with its emphasis on formal equality, the absence of coercion and political participation in electoral processes. There are, however, a number of problems arising from this view of citizenship – and the social figure it generates – which are related to the shifting character of the concept and its obscuring of the inequalities which lie beneath the surface of the formal equality all citizens share in law. Yuval-Davis (1997) has pointed to the shifting character of citizenship when she says that it:

> has been constructed in different ways in different societies and has undergone historical shifts within the same state and society. It has been subject to contesting ideologies from the left and the right, and used as an inclusive and exclusive organizing principle, as a political mobilization tool and as a means of the depoliticization of the population. Also, in spite of its universalist terminology it has been applied differently to different segments of the population in each country.
>
> (Yuval-Davis, 1997, p.68)

What features does Yuval-Davis suggest are indicative of citizenship's shifting character?

Taylor (1996) has raised similar concerns in explicit reference to the power relations which are masked by the formal equality among citizens:

> Indeed, the liberal tradition of citizenship, resting on an abstract notion of rights and an appeal to *universalism,* has ignored the particular reality of power. In this context, social relations of power are seen as taking historically varying forms, but most notably those associated with class, gender and 'race'. These historically specific power relations have undermined attempts to realize the liberal ideal of citizenship ...
>
> (Taylor, 1996, pp.156–7)

The implication of these arguments is that the idea of citizenship is full of ambiguity, subject to shifting definition according to time and place, whilst the 'rights' which accrue to diverse citizens depend upon the distribution of social power and the inequalities which this distribution reflects and produces. In part the ambiguities carried by the term citizenship and the inequalities it masks are themselves a reflection of the terminological conflation of two distinct and

liberalism

107

contradictory principles, as Silverman (1996) has pointed out. He notes that the liberal conception of the abstract citizen contains within it both the notion of 'the civil' and that of 'the civic', which, following Leca (1991), he distinguishes in the following way:

the civil
the civic

> The first of these, the civil, refers to the private individual and is underscored by the principles of liberalism, the market and inegalitarianism; the second of these, the civic, refers to the individual who is part of a community of rights and is underscored by the principles of intervention, egalitarianism and solidarity.
>
> (Silverman, 1996, p.147)

The notion of citizenship therefore contains within it a number of contradictory discourses about the relation between the individual and the state which can be expressed as a series of oppositions – between the collective and the individual, rights and responsibilities, and equality and inequality. These dimensions, or fields of potential tension and opposition, were at the heart of debates in the UK about citizenship both at the end of the Second World War and on the cusp of the twenty-first century. In both periods the link between 'the citizen', the state and social welfare provided the axis around which these questions were addressed and struggled over. This was the issue which most concerned T.H. Marshall and, bearing in mind the points raised above, it is to this that we now turn.

ACTIVITY 3.1

Before proceeding to the next section, stop for a moment and think about the ways in which you think of yourself as a citizen. For example, what *rights* do you think you have as a result of your citizenship? What, if any, *duties* do you have? Do you think of yourself as 'belonging' to a national community? If so, is it the same one as the nation-state in which you reside?

COMMENT

You may have included in your list of rights things such as the right to free speech or the right to vote. You might also have thought about the right to freedom of movement, freedom to practise whatever religion you choose, and the right to work. In terms of duties, you may have included the duty to obey the law and pay taxes. These two duties were certainly the most commonly listed by those consulted by the All Party Commission on Citizenship (HMSO, 1990, p.6). You may also have included as a duty the responsibility to provide for yourself and your dependants. What about the rights associated with welfare services – did you list any of these? Again, the Commission found that rights to a minimum standard of living and access to medical care, work and education were at the top of the list of those consulted. In asking yourself the question about national belonging, it may be that you answered this in terms of your legal nationality, but it is important to recognize that a sense of national belonging may be a part of an identity even if no recognized state exists which can bestow citizenship status upon you. Palestine and Kurdistan are two such examples, and what about Wales, Scotland and Northern Ireland? Similarly, many people live in different nation-states to those which accord them their citizenship status, and some of these will have dual nationality.

3 Citizenship and welfare: T.H. Marshall

For many who displayed a renewed interest in the relationship between social welfare and citizenship in the last part of the twentieth century the work of T.H. Marshall some 40 years earlier provided the starting-point for their discussions. In part this was due to the fact that Marshall put the relation between the citizen, the state and social welfare at the centre of analysis. He did this by suggesting that citizenship comprised three aspects. Thus, for him, citizenship should be thought of as divided into its civil element, its political element and its social element: as the following, originally published in 1950, makes clear:

> The *civil* element is composed of the rights necessary for individual freedom – liberty of the person, freedom of speech, thought and faith, the right to own property and to conclude valid contracts, and the right to justice. The last is of a different order from the others, because it is the right to defend and assert all one's rights on terms of equality with others and by due process of law. This shows us that the institutions most directly associated with civil rights are the courts of justice. By the *political* element I mean the right to participate in the exercise of political power, as a member of a body invested with political authority or as an elector of the members of such a body. The corresponding institutions are parliament and councils of local government. By the *social* element I mean the whole range from the right to a modicum of economic welfare and security to the right to share to the full in the social heritage and to live the life of a civilized being according to the standards prevailing in the society. The institutions most closely connected with it are the education system and the social services.
>
> (Marshall, 1996, p.8)

According to Marshall, these three aspects of citizenship were the result of an evolutionary process, with each element, though overlapping, being associated with the eighteenth, nineteenth and twentieth centuries respectively. As such, *social citizenship*, and its direct link to welfare institutions, was a feature of twentieth-century democratic societies and made citizenship a profoundly *relational* concept which constructed a particular version of the relation between the state and its citizens.

To what extent do you think there is a correspondence between Marshall's civil element and the definition of the civil made by Silverman given in section 2?

Fundamental to Marshall's analysis of citizenship was the relationship between social welfare and social class and the ways in which citizenship could mediate this relation. In particular he was concerned to reconcile two incompatible principles or trends, each of which was characteristic of the modern democratic capitalist state – the equality of citizens and the inequalities of class. Central to this was his conception of the relation and tension between the rights of citizenship and the necessity of the free market economy. Or, to put it another way, citizenship rights inhibit the inegalitarian tendencies of capitalism, but the market, and economic inequality, are necessary for the production of wealth and the preservation of political rights. Let us begin to explore this potentially conflicting relation by considering the way in which Marshall posits the tension between the equality of citizenship and the inequality of class.

Read through Extract 3.1 which is taken from Marshall's 1950 essay 'Citizenship and social class'. As you do so, make a note of the following:

■ how Marshall defines citizenship;

■ in what ways he sees it as an equalizing principle;

■ how he defines class;

■ why class is a system of inequality.

Extract 3.1 Marshall: 'Equalizing the unequal?'

Citizenship is a status bestowed on those who are full members of a community. All who possess the status are equal with respect to the rights and duties with which the status is endowed. There is no universal principle that determines what those rights and duties shall be, but societies in which citizenship is a developing institution create an image of an ideal citizenship against which achievement can be measured and towards which aspiration can be directed. The urge forward along the path thus plotted is an urge towards a fuller measure of equality, an enrichment of the stuff of which the status is made and an increase in the number of those on whom the status is bestowed. Social class, on the other hand, is a system of inequality. And it too, like citizenship, can be based on a set of ideals, beliefs and values. It is therefore reasonable to expect that the impact of citizenship on social class should take the form of a conflict between opposing principles. ...

It is at this point that a closer scrutiny of social class becomes necessary. ... there is one broad distinction between two different types of class which is particularly relevant ... In the first of these class is based on a hierarchy of status, and the difference between one class and another is expressed in terms of legal rights and of established customs which have the essential binding character of law. ... differences between social levels are not differences in standard of living, because there is no common standard by which they can be measured. Nor are there any rights ... which all share in common. ... The rights with which the general status of citizenship was invested were extracted from the hierarchical status system of social class, robbing it of its essential substance. The equality implicit in the concept of citizenship, even though limited in content, undermined the inequality of the class system, which was in principle a total inequality. National justice and a law common to all must inevitably weaken and eventually destroy class justice, and personal freedom, as universal birthright, must drive out serfdom. No subtle argument is needed to show that citizenship is incompatible with medieval feudalism.

Social class of the second type is not so much an institution in its own right as a by-product of other institutions. ... Class differences are not established and defined by the laws and customs of the society (in the medieval sense of the phrase), but emerge from the interplay of a variety of factors related to the institutions of property and education and the structure of the national economy. Class cultures dwindle to a minimum, so that it becomes possible, though admittedly not wholly satisfactory, to measure the different levels of economic welfare by reference to a common standard of living. ...

It is true that class still functions. Social inequality is regarded as necessary and purposeful. It provides the incentive to effort and designs the distribution of power. But there is no overall pattern of inequality, in which an appropriate value is attached, a priori, to each social level. Inequality therefore, though necessary, may become excessive.

(Marshall, 1996, pp.18–20)

COMMENT

This extract makes it immediately clear that, for Marshall, citizenship is a status accorded to people who can claim full membership of a community – though it is not clear what criteria are used to accord such membership. At a basic level, citizenship acts as an equalizing principle because its benefits – that is, the rights and duties which are attached to it – are applied equally to all who belong to the community and can claim the status. It is also an equalizing principle because the status is accorded to an ever increasing number of people.

In contrast, class is a system of inequality. But to understand why this is so we have to look at how Marshall defines class. He distinguishes between two sorts of class system. On the one hand, he identifies a class system based on the formal ascription of a certain place within a hierarchy of social positions. In this sort of class system these positions are fixed – denying any possibility of social mobility – and they are about status and not standard of living. Examples of this sort of class system would be serfdom or caste systems. On the other hand, there is a class system more characteristic of capitalist societies (though some capitalist societies will have both forms co-existing). This second system of class derives from the workings of the economy and other social systems, such as education. It is not a closed system and mobility across class boundaries is possible.

In the contexts of both these systems of class, though especially the latter, the equalizing effect of citizenship becomes deepened. Thus, for Marshall, citizenship acts in this way because it pushes at the boundaries of the former and moderates the excessive effects of the latter. It does this by according a universal principle of protected rights alongside the inequalities generated by the economic system.

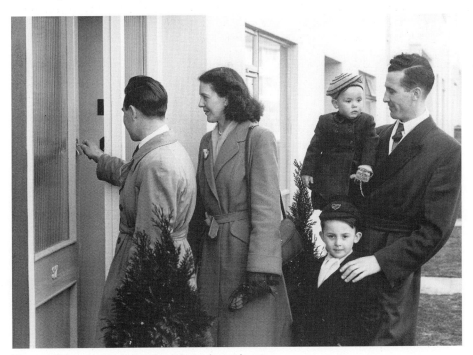

The social democratic citizen: the right to decent housing

It should be clear that in this context the social aspect of citizenship has an especially important role to play in ameliorating the excesses of class inequality. The social element of citizenship can act in this way because it provides the 'common standard of living' against which the claim to participation in the social heritage is measured. Thus the incorporation of the social element into citizenship has meant that the aspiration for the diminution of class-based social inequalities came to the fore. However, this was not because what matters is the equalization of *incomes*, but rather because the object was an equalization of *status* among individuals and general participation in the social life of the society. Extract 3.2, taken from the same essay as Extract 3.1, shows how Marshall thought of this.

Extract 3.2 Marshall: 'Broadening equality: status not income'

[Until the end of the nineteenth century] [s]ocial rights were at a minimum and were not woven into the fabric of citizenship. The common purpose of statutory and voluntary effort was to abate the nuisance of poverty without disturbing the pattern of inequality of which poverty was the most obviously unpleasant consequence.

A new period opened at the end of the nineteenth century ... It saw the first big advance in social rights, and this involved significant changes in the egalitarian principles expressed in citizenship. ...

These aspirations [for the diminution of inequality] have in part been met by incorporating social rights in the status of citizenship and thus creating a universal right to real income which is not proportionate to the market value of the claimant. Class-abatement is still the aim of social rights, but it has acquired a new meaning. It is no longer merely an attempt to abate the obvious nuisance of destitution in the lowest ranks of society. It has assumed the guise of action modifying the whole pattern of social inequality. ... It is therefore important to consider whether any such ultimate aim is implicit in the nature of this development, or whether ... there are natural limits to the contemporary drive towards greater social and economic equality. ...

The extension of the social services is not primarily a means of equalizing incomes. ... What matters is that there is a general enrichment of the concrete substance of civilised life, a general reduction of risk and insecurity, an equalisation between the more and the less fortunate at all levels – between the healthy and the sick, the employed and the unemployed, the old and the active, the bachelor and the father of a large family. Equalisation is not so much between *classes* as between *individuals* within a population which is now treated for this purpose as though it were one class. Equality of status is more important than equality of income.

The unified civilisation which makes social inequalities acceptable, and threatens to make them economically functionless, is achieved by a progressive divorce between real and money incomes. This is, of course, explicit in the major social services, such as health and education, which give benefits in kind without any *ad hoc* payment. In scholarships and legal aid, prices scaled to money incomes keep real income relatively constant, in so far as it is affected by these particular needs. Rent restriction, combined with security of tenure, achieves a similar result by different means. ... The advantages obtained by having a larger money income do not disappear, but they are confined to a limited area of consumption.

(Marshall, 1996, pp.27–8, 33, 47, emphasis added)

For those familiar with the main principles and objectives of the welfare state which was inaugurated by the Beveridge reforms of the mid to late 1940s (see, for example, **Cochrane, 1998; Hughes, 1998**), it is clear from this extract that Marshall can also be considered as one of the architects of the welfare state. Thus, in his conception of citizenship, its relation to a capitalist system of social organization, and, more importantly, his vision of the relationship between the state, the individual and welfare benefits and services, Marshall shared many of the aims and visions of Beveridge and Keynes. Another way of thinking about this is to regard these three as influencing the formation of the 'common sense' about welfare at this time. Despite this, in Extract 3.2 Marshall collapses the collectivity of class into the individual, and thus provides us with an illustration of the conflation of the 'civil' with the 'civic' which we noted earlier as common to many conceptions of citizenship. Nevertheless, he retains the notion of the welfare state as an equalizing set of institutions and services because it constitutes the mechanisms through which equality of citizenship status is given substance.

Central to this are the redistributive effects of the social wage in the form of welfare services which Marshall takes to mean: 'the whole apparatus that includes social security, education, public health, the medical services, factory legislation, the right to strike, and all the other rights and legitimate expectations which are attached to modern democratic citizenship' (Marshall, 1981a, p.81). For Marshall, then, welfare and citizenship are inseparable. In this context he implies a shift in the locus of inequality away from inequalities in the money wage and rights of citizens towards those inequalities which properly exist between different areas of welfare. Marshall indicates what he means by this shift in the locus of inequality in a contrast he draws between the system of legal aid and that of the health service. Let us take a moment to see how he makes the distinction between these two services and how, therefore, he legitimates the inequalities which may result from such a distinction. The key to the distinction is the question of subjective or objective assessments of value and need (see **Langan, 1998,** on the social construction of need). Thus in the case of legal aid (for civil law cases) he argues that their value is subjective because it is something which can only be determined by the parties to the litigation. This he contrasts with health, 'where the seriousness of the disease and the nature of the treatment required can be objectively assessed with very little reference to the importance the patient attaches to it' (Marshall, 1996, p.29). Citizenship thus becomes a status of entitlement and a means for articulating and managing a field of competing rights – that is, economic, political and social rights – and ensuring social cohesion.

How was the term 'articulates' defined at the beginning of this chapter?

Citizenship, or the equality of rights it generates, becomes an integrative process counteracting the tendencies towards social division and conflict generated by the economic system. By now, then, it should be clear that, for Marshall, inequality was not in itself a problem. His project was to find an acceptable balance between the forces for inequality and those for equality. He also thought it desirable to distinguish between areas of the welfare state where greater degrees of inequality were acceptable and those where this was not the case, as the example of his contrast between legal aid and the health service illustrates.

However, it may be that more deep-rooted and excluding forms of inequality result from this conception of citizenship and, in sections 5 and 6, I consider two areas where this is the case. At this point I want to explore a little further the implications of Marshall's attempt to shift inequality to *areas* of welfare to see whether or not it leads to forms of inequality between formally equal categories of *person*. One way to approach this is to consider how he elaborates his distinction between areas of welfare in terms of the question of the *duties* which are a part of citizenship. On this Marshall argues that the meeting of certain social rights (understood as broadly defined welfare rights) is simultaneously the meeting of *duties* by the individual citizen. He clearly states his position in relation to education and health:

> For education is not only something to which every citizen has a right; it is a process by which citizens are made. As such it is something that every society must promote in its own interest ... Education is of such vital importance for the health and prosperity of a nation, that it is regarded as something of which the individual has a *duty* to avail himself, to the extent that his natural abilities warrant ...
>
> It is just as important for a society to have a healthy population as to have an educated one, so the right to health, like the right to education, is blended with duties. Public health is in large measure a form of public discipline, and the element of obligation spreads from environmental to personal health, from one's duty to one's neighbours to one's duty to one's dependants and one's duty to oneself. Health regulations, health visitors and health education are there to promote welfare by stressing a duty even more than a right ...
>
> (Marshall, 1981b, pp.90–1)

Thus citizenship constructs a mutuality between rights and duties. However, this balance or mutuality is not distributed equally among all who might make the claim to citizenship and it is here that we can begin to pursue the substantive inequalities which result from the Marshallian view of citizenship.

This is most clearly discernible in connection with what Marshall refers to as the moral dimension and his insistence on the importance of a parallel system of discretionary rights to welfare alongside those (such as health, education, employment) which must be universal. Here we can see the potential for the construction of a second-class citizenship.

ACTIVITY 3.3

Extract 3.3, taken from a subsequent essay by Marshall entitled 'The right to welfare', illustrates further the distinctions Marshall drew between different sites of welfare. Read through this extract carefully and, as you do so, make a note of your responses to the following questions:

1   How does Marshall balance the social and individual dimensions of the right to education and health?

2   What evidence is there of a potential for differentiation leading to the construction of subordinated (or second-class) welfare subjects?

3   On what basis does he posit a distinction between social rights and moral rights?

Extract 3.3 Marshall: 'The limits of "rights"'

The modern rights to education and health are ... not merely recognised by all as being social in origin, but are part of the mechanism by which the individual is absorbed into society (not isolated from it) and which simultaneously draws upon and contributes to its collective welfare.

The case of the welfare services, in the technical administrative sense [that is, personal social services] is different. It cannot be said that society needs happy old people in the same way that it needs a healthy and educated population. Nor would it suffer any grave loss if the mentally handicapped were not assisted (at considerable cost in time and money) to make the most of their limited capacities. The motive that inspires the services rendered to these people is compassion rather than interest. And though compassion … may create a right, having almost the force of law, to minimal subsistence, it cannot establish the same kind of right to the benefit of services which are continuously striving to extend the limits of the possible, and to replace the minimum by the optimum. So this particular right to welfare is bound to be more dependent than the others for its driving and sustaining force on the fact that it is a moral right. … Furthermore, those in need of these welfare services are minority groups, set apart from the general body of normal citizens by their disabilities. The principle of universality which is a characteristic feature of the modern rights of citizenship does not apply, and the right cannot be reinforced, as in the case of education and health, by a corresponding duty to exercise it. The most one can say is that the handicapped have a moral duty to try to overcome their misfortunes as far as in them lies.

(Marshall, 1981b, pp.91–2)

COMMENT

Here we see again the mutuality between social rights and individual duties. Importantly, the balance between the social and the individual is achieved via the integrative effects of citizenship rights to welfare. However, if these rights have a general integrative effect, the distinctions Marshall draws between different areas of welfare also make for the potential to construct some citizens as second class. This is achieved in two stages. First, by suggesting that, unlike education and health, society derives no general benefits from the personal social services; and, second, by saying that those who do have a need for such services only have a second-order

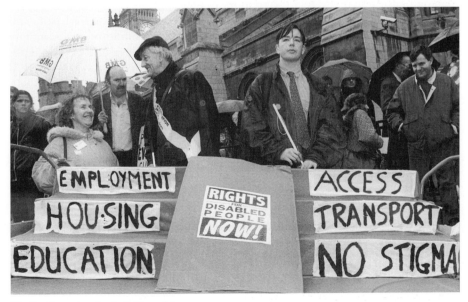

Challenging subordinated citizenship

115

right (for minimal subsistence) which derives from compassion (moral) not collective (social) self-interest. In this way Marshall both distinguishes the bases of moral and social rights and constructs differentiated categories of citizen or subordinated welfare subjects (see **Lewis, 1998a,b**). Thus we can see that the notion of citizenship is a constructed category which, despite its suggestion of formal equality, contains its own boundaries of belonging and outsiderness.

■ ■ ■

Marshall, then, gives us rights and redistribution, social integration and formal equality. He also gives us inequality and exclusion by placing a normative figure at the centre of his idea of citizenship, which, though he never specifically defined this as such, we came to understand as being the white, able-bodied and breadwinner male (see section 6; and **Hughes, 1998**). In later sections we will turn our attention to some of these issues of inequality; in the section which follows, however, we will look at one example of the re-emergence of a discourse of citizenship in late twentieth century.

4   The re-emergence of citizenship as a category of political articulation

We left Marshall at the point where he talked about citizenship as carrying duties, as well as rights, and that, whilst it was a status, it was also something which was learnt. In making this suggestion about the learned character of citizenship, Marshall echoed ideas about citizenship which were present in many debates about state-organized education in the early part of the twentieth century (see, for example, **McCoy, 1998**). In a similar way we can see examples of the link made between formal education and citizenship by official sources in the late twentieth century. However, one of the main points of divergence between Marshall's approach and that found in more recent publications and debates is that citizenship, and the rights it accords, has been disarticulated from the objective of redistribution and rearticulated to forms of voluntary-sector activity (which Marshall noted as a hallmark of the nineteenth century). This later approach – or, properly stated, this re-emergent approach – is exemplified in the report of the All Party Parliamentary Commission on Citizenship (HMSO, 1990). As such, it provides a way of thinking about why and in what ways the notion of citizenship re-entered the political arena at a time when the social democratic welfare state had undergone radical restructuring.

ACTIVITY 3.4

Extract 3.4 is taken from the report of the All Party Parliamentary Commission on Citizenship. As you read through it, think about:

■ the social changes the authors of the report identify as providing the context for the re-emergence of citizenship as an important idea and status in the last decade of the twentieth century;

■ whether the civil or the civic is foregrounded in their approach as represented here;

■ the relative importance given to rights and duties.

Extract 3.4 All Party Parliamentary Commission on Citizenship: 'Encouraging citizenship'

The theme of this Report is the separate role of individuals as citizens within the political or public community, and the rules that govern it. We believe that citizenship is one of the most important concepts of modern political struggle and social development. …

Our society is passing through a period of change and we are concerned that without our realising it, we could lose some of the benefits of living in the relatively free and open society which we have inherited. The status and entitlements of all individuals is affected by the United Kingdom's membership of the European Communities and changing relationship with the Commonwealth. Since the war, Britain has been transformed into a multi-racial society. At the same time, shifts in the income, life style, nature of work and demographic balance of the population are affecting people's expectations, traditional arrangements for working life, retirement and care in the community.

Furthermore, the individual's role as a consumer and the responsibility of Government to safeguard freedom of choice has been reasserted over the last decade. In parallel, the scope, role, finance, management and accountability of public services has been contested. … Citizenship … is a cultural achievement, a gift from history, which can be lost or destroyed. The Commission's purpose in publishing this Report is to propose practical ways in which our participatory arrangements can be strengthened so that they remain efficient rather than simply dignified, or ceremonial, parts of the constitution.

The challenge to our society in the late twentieth century is to create conditions where all who wish can become actively involved, can understand and participate, can influence, persuade, campaign and whistleblow, and in the making of decisions can work together for the mutual good. We deliberately did not … confine our attention to formal structures alone, for civil, political and social entitlements and services are not delivered solely through official institutions. We considered the numerous forms of independent and voluntary contribution to society and its citizens, for they too play an important part. …

Having considered the many factors described in the Report … we drew up a series of recommendations for action. …

Recommendations

Learning to be a citizen

[The Commission recommends:]

1. … that the study and experience of citizenship should be a part of every young person's education from the earliest years of schooling and continuing into the post-school years within further and higher education and the youth service, whether in state or private sector schools, and irrespective of the course of study being followed. …

3. … that every school governing body should request that a strategy should be developed and monitored for incorporating citizenship studies across the curriculum; …

4. … that evidence of activities undertaken as part of learning citizenship skills across the curriculum should be included in a student's Record of Achievement. …

7. … that institutions in the higher education sector should formulate explicit selection policies and consider how most appropriately to take into account evidence of a candidate's citizenship activities.

8.   ... that each local education authority reviews the range and type of support available for community work and citizenship activities, particularly within the youth service and adult education.

9.   ... that the judiciary, civil service, teachers, doctors and nurses, local government officers, the police and the armed forces should have specific training on the entitlements and duties of citizens and the corresponding obligations of public institutions ...

Public services and the voluntary sector

12.   ... that a floor of adequate social entitlements should be maintained, monitored and improved when possible by central government, with the aim of enabling every citizen to live the life of a civilised human being according to the standards prevailing in society.

13.   ... that central government should complement the investigations into the extent of volunteer activity and the work of the voluntary sector now being carried out ... by co-ordinating a public review, which would determine:

(a)   the boundaries between statutory and voluntary responsibilities in the public services on a sector by sector basis

(b)   the boundaries between the roles of professionals and auxiliary workers and those of volunteers in publicly funded services

(c)   ways of ensuring efficient and effective use of public funds through a cost-benefit analysis of the potential contribution of volunteers to service agencies

(d)   guidelines for the involvement of under-represented groups ...

(HMSO, 1990, pp.xv–xvi, xviii–xix)

COMMENT

A list of social changes provides the starting-point for the authors' argument that citizenship is a key social and political question for the UK in the late twentieth century. This list includes: entry into the European Union and the changed relationship with the Commonwealth; shifts in lifestyle, labour markets and working patterns; altered patterns of care, demographic changes and the 'multi-racial' character of the UK. What is particularly striking about this extract is that these changes provide the context for the discussion of citizenship because, the authors suggest, they could result in the established benefits of citizenship being undermined. *Why* this might be the case is, however, not clear. What *is* clear is that the authors imply that these changes necessitate the implementation of a series of mechanisms through which to reconnect disparate segments of the population to an organic whole. As such, the extract constructs a particular vision of 'the people' now and the lines of connection among them in the future, and thus advocates a particular position within the field of competing contestations over the future relationship between the state and the individual.

At the same time the authors construct an ambiguous mix between the civil and the civic. In section 2 a distinction was drawn between these two dimensions and it is worth taking a moment to remind yourself of this. Here it is clear that the civil – in the form of the rights of the individual to exercise their freedom of choice as a consumer and have this guaranteed by government – is foregrounded. On the other hand, the civic – in the sense of participation in the political life of the community – is also evident. However, this is so in a context in which the more solidaristic and egalitarian rights, which have been associated with the social democratic welfare state in which the state guarantees those mechanisms of redistribution, are downplayed. Thus rights and duties, in this extract, are most commonly expressed in terms of the right and duty to participate in forms of voluntary-sector, charitable and philanthropic activity. Such participation, in fact, is presented as the hallmark of 'good' citizenship and it is this which should be promoted in the education system and elsewhere. Indeed, the authors of the report claim that their approach is in keeping with that of the 'British people', since they 'have adopted as a yardstick for contemporary re-evaluation of citizenship an analysis which, so far as we can judge, corresponds to the perceptions of the British people today' (HMSO, 1990, p.xv). Who makes up the 'British people' and how the report's authors come to know their views is less clear, but the approach exemplified here does allow us to see the ways in which the figure of the citizen has been reworked in a manner which facilitates a new way of imagining the relationship between the state, welfare services and individuals/communities. As such, the extract provides a clear example of the reworking of the Marshallian conception of citizenship which was at the heart of the post Second World War welfare state. However, if this social democratic figure of the citizen has been reworked, what should replace it has been much contested and in the following section attention is turned to two opposing approaches to this issue.

■ ■ ■

5   Markets, personal autonomy and 'the public sphere'

Whilst it is clear that part of the restructuring of the welfare state since the 1980s has carried with it an attempt to reformulate the relationship between the state and the individual, the direction this reformulation should take has been open to much contestation. From the discussion so far it should be clear that, at least since the 1950s, the figure of the citizen has occupied a central place in the articulation of a set of connections expressed as state–individual–welfare services. This should be kept in mind as you consider how this set of connections is constructed in Extracts 3.5 and 3.6 given in this section. A feature common to both the 'imaginative acts' presented here is the way in which the authors connect citizenship to questions of autonomy. Taken as one example of a debate between positions which can broadly be described as coming from within the New Right (in the first instance) and the Left (in the second instance), they illustrate two positions on the question of whether state-organized welfare promotes or strangles individual autonomy. As such, they re-pose the question of the citizen of welfare in terms of the structures and processes required to promote such autonomy. Importantly, the issues raised move away from any simple either/or dichotomy of the market or the state and instead focus on the form of citizenship best suited to the production and distribution of symbolic and material goods.

Extracts 3.5 and 3.6 are taken from work by David Green, on the one hand, and David Purdy, on the other. Chapter 2 has already considered the work of Green, so his approach will not be entirely new to you. He is concerned to promote what he calls 'civic capitalism' in which he formulates a mechanism for the production and distribution of welfare services outside of that associated with the social democratic welfare state. Indeed, Green subscribes to the view that this form of welfare has created welfare dependency and strangled individual enterprise and creativity. Purdy is also concerned to formulate a new way of connecting individuals to welfare goods and services but he does so in a way which re-establishes and strengthens the role of the state in this process. This is via the payment of what he calls a Citizen's, or Basic, Income. In this way Purdy considers some of the issues concerning class inequalities which we began to consider above. The continued focus on class is important since the persistence and increase in poverty and other forms of class-derived inequality which occurred in the 1980s and 1990s ensure that class remains a central aspect of debates about citizenship.

More broadly, the two extracts are useful because they allow us to consider further two other issues. The first is the obvious one of enabling us to contrast competing constructions of future welfare belongings, entitlements and duties – or what we might call the social and symbolic relations of welfare. Second, they allow us to think about these issues in more abstract or conceptual terms. Specifically, they help us to think about the connection between the individual and social aspects of citizenship to which Held (1991) referred and which were discussed in section 2; they are also a means by which to illustrate how 'citizenship' is one way of constructing a national popular. This second set of issues may appear difficult to grasp at this point, but they should become clearer as you read through Extracts 3.5 and 3.6. To help you with this you should work through them in two stages – each time reading with a different set of questions in mind.

<hr>

ACTIVITY 3.5(A)

Set 1 Reading for contrasting positions
Read Extracts 3.5 and 3.6. In this first reading think about and make a note of the differences between:

- the role accorded to the individual;

- the role accorded to the sphere of the 'public';

- how the authors place the 'market' in their respective visions of a welfare future;

- why each author dismisses economic growth as a *sufficient* condition for the transformation of welfare relations;

- the ways in which each extract makes a moral argument.

<hr>

Extract 3.5 Imaginative act 1. Green: 'Re-energizing civil society: a proposal'

Here are some possible means of developing a new approach aimed at restoring the dependent poor to independent citizenship. The underlying assumption is that practical help is superior to mere almsgiving, whether by charity or the state. Sending giro cheques is too easy. Real caring means time and trouble, not mere cash support. The purpose … is to give the able-bodied poor the opportunity to put something back, not only to spend.

The chief danger to be avoided is the 'crowding out' effect of the welfare state. As state welfare has grown so it has squeezed out voluntary associations and diminished the spirit of personal responsibility on which a vibrant civil society rests. …

The policies that might follow from this approach fall into three groups: (1) policies aimed at economic growth; (2) the removal of public-policy obstacles to family or personal advancement, particularly high taxes; and (3) a focus on personal independence.

1. Economic growth

The focus on individual conduct and morals is indispensable to success, but on its own will not be sufficient. Economic growth is a necessary, but not sufficient, pre-condition for the creation of opportunities to escape from poverty. Economic growth depends in large measure on the energy and ingenuity of private citizens, but unwise fiscal and monetary policies can all too easily cancel out human endeavour. Government, therefore, has a responsibility to create an economic framework consistent with liberty.

2. Removal of public-policy impediments

Some public policies ... narrow opportunities to escape from poverty. Particular culprits are high taxes on incomes and savings, and the inadequate integration of taxes and benefits. A comprehensive reform programme is necessary to remove the impediments which make it more difficult for the poor to advance by their own endeavours. ... all proposals [for] reform ... should be subject to 'independence impact assessments' to guage their effect on efforts by individuals to escape from poverty by their own endeavours.

These assessments should include examination of impediments to labour mobility ...

Taxation policy should be subject to especially close scrutiny. Tax thresholds should be raised to allow workers to keep more of their earnings. Child tax allowances should be restored and the married person's allowance increased substantially as part of a general raising of tax thresholds and in order to bolster the traditional two-parent family. The mutual support of the family still remains the best foundation for independence. ...

3. Personal independence planning

There are many reasons for unemployment. ...

Here, I am concerned about people who are unemployed because they lack the skills and motivation to help themselves out of their predicament. We are not succeeding in helping this group and there is a need for new policies aimed at assisting such individuals. Focusing on individually-tailored help and advice is highly desirable but ... it seems unlikely that a government department can ever be the best instrument for such work. An alternative approach would be to transfer programmes intended to help particular individuals back into the workforce to private care associations, which would be charged with devising an 'independence plan' for each person. ...

Conclusion

... The battle against collectivist economics has led us to over-estimate the importance of markets in maintaining liberty and to neglect both the moral dimension of a free society and the corruption of law making by politics.

Civic capitalists, therefore, hope for three main changes. First, they advocate constitutional reform to re-establish the impartiality of law by separating the process of law making from the implementation of political programmes. ...

Second, we must refresh our understanding of the moral case against the welfare state. Much of what we call the welfare state should be returned to civil society, especially education and health care, not to save money, nor to improve the 'targeting' of benefits, and not even to improve efficiency, but above all to prevent the suppression of opportunities for bringing out the best in people through service of others. The state should maintain a safety net below which no one should fall, but any help beyond the state minimum should be primarily private in order to widen the scope for individual generosity and service of others … [that is] to increase the scope for civil society, … the realm of free choice and conscience as opposed to the realm of government command.

Third, civic capitalists hope to encourage debate about the moral climate that makes freedom possible. Above all, we need a new ethos of social solidarity which rests, not on income transfers, but on mutual consideration for others and a strong sense of personal responsibility.

(Green, 1993, pp.147, 149–50, 152–3)

Extract 3.6 Imaginative act 2. Purdy: 'A citizen's income'

The rival vision [to that of the neo-liberal variant of the New Right] of the future is no less ambitious and no less concerned with personal freedom. But it appeals to widely held notions of social justice and seeks to reinvent the concept of social citizenship. … it draws on both liberal and socialist traditions of thought, and since it rests on values to which large numbers of people in our society would assent – at least on reflection, if not without question – it could, in time and if correctly handled, win the support of a broad social and political coalition.

At the heart of this attempt to reformulate and revitalize the social rights of citizenship is the idea of Citizen's Income [CI]. CI differs from all existing social transfers in that it is payable:

i) to individuals rather than families or households;

ii) irrespective of income from other sources;

iii) without requiring any past or present work performance, or any test of willingness to seek paid work or accept jobs if they are offered. …

… BI [Basic Income which is the other name Purdy uses] would transform people's options in the labour market, with potentially far-reaching consequences for economy and society. No one knows how people would reallocate their energies, skills and time if their basic living costs were unconditionally guaranteed. Clearly, much would depend on the wider stance of public policy, interacting with private choice. But it strains credulity to suppose that BI would make no difference whatsoever to labour-force participation rates, the duration and pattern of working time, the sexual division of labour and other structural aspects of social reproduction. …

Of course, until Basic Income capitalism is actually tried, we can only speculate about its dynamics. Exactly the same was true of mass democracy prior to the extension of the suffrage. But speculation need not be unbridled, and is, indeed, indispensable in a context where it makes no sense to assume that the future will be just like the past. … In any case, beliefs about the limits of social possibility are themselves a factor in determining the course of events, regardless of whether they are, in some sense, well-founded. …

More generally, if the ethos of social citizenship takes hold, people may be less inclined to take a narrow, sectional view of their interests and more receptive to the claims of wider moral communities, including those of their fellow citizens …

It would … be unwise to expect economic growth alone to ease the transition to a 'full' Basic Income. 'Growthist' strategies ignore the cultural dimension of social citizenship. Any sensible definition of poverty has to be culturally relative. Hence, BI scales will tend to rise in proportion to per capita GDP [gross domestic product]. But this implies that a 'full' BI will *never* be viable without a change in taxpayers' collective willingness to shoulder the 'burden'. Thus, whether and how far society travels from welfare-state capitalism to Basic Income capitalism and beyond, will depend less on the rate of economic growth and more on the state of social relations.

… The public realm

Social policy involves the provision or purchase of social services as well as the funding and management of social transfers. …

In a state which respects the moral equality of persons, the logic of citizenship is egalitarian, whereas markets have an inherent tendency to produce or perpetuate disparities of social condition. …

… all actual market economies [as opposed to ideal typical ones], to varying degrees, are marked by deep-rooted and long-lasting divisions of gender, class, race and ethnicity. … some of these divisions predate the rise of capitalism and the spread of market relations – by millennia in the case of gender. This does not prevent them from continuing to distort the distribution of income, work and power. And typically, though not invariably, these same divisions also shape the pattern of society's principle distributive conflicts. …

[In contrast to this pull of the market] where citizenship entails rights and duties which are shared in common by all, it can, in principle, correct the 'spontaneous' lean of the social structure. If this potential is to be realized, however, citizenship must become an active force in public affairs, not just the source of a passive, recipient right to the means of subsistence.

As a school of active citizenship, the combination of full commodification with a 'full' Basic Income looks distinctly unpromising. For one thing, money alone cannot correct structural disadvantage. But more importantly, if public services are privatized, and social policy is reduced to the redistribution of purchasing power, then apart from their strictly financial rights and responsibilities as beneficiaries and taxpayers, people will only ever experience each other as market participants: that is, as traders, customers, suppliers, consumers, employers, employees, third parties and so on.

… the pursuit of self-interest – or to be more precise, the pursuit of *commercial* self-interest – is a powerful force for material progress. But it is singularly ill-adapted to the pursuit of social justice. …

Citizen's Income is likely to flourish under a strong and expansive public realm based on active partnership between state and civil society. To see why, consider how CI is to be financed. In principle, taxes could be levied on the income, expenditure or wealth of persons; on the profits, sales or payrolls of enterprises; or on some combination of all of these. But the choice of a tax base is not just a matter of making ends meet: it is likely to have profound consequences for the way people perceive and pursue their interests. The preceding argument suggests that a good tax-transfer system is one which promotes active citizenship and economic democracy, enhancing society's capacity to handle distributive conflict without recourse to either brute coercion or the impersonal discipline of the market. …

There is little hope of achieving this goal if the government attempts to steer the economy by remote control, setting the parameters of the tax-transfer system and leaving private agents in civil society to work out their own salvation. ...

In a 'Basic Income Democracy' government would deliberately and regularly seek to foster public debate about tax-transfer policy by issuing a standing invitation to all sectional interests to identify policy options, explore their implications and argue the case for pursuing one option rather than another.

Sectional claims and counter-claims would not disappear. Nor would this be desirable. But sectional interest groups would be obliged to frame and justify their claims in ways that took account of people's shared identity as citizens. Conversely, the policy-making process would acquire a sharper focus, and citizens would be better placed to make genuine choices about their collective, long-term future, giving due weight to the respective claims of social justice, economic growth and ecological sustainability.

(Purdy, 1994, pp.33, 41–5)

New Labour and Green: is there a commonality of view?

'... redistribution of cash from rich to poor which others artificially choose as their own limited definition of egalitarianism. ... The people we are concerned about ... will not have their long-term problems addressed by an extra pound a week on their benefits ... we must concentrate effort on helping individuals who can escape their situation to do so, in the knowledge that personal skills and employment are the most effective anti-poverty policy in the long run.'

Peter Mandelson, Minister without Portfolio, speech to the Fabian Society, 14 August 1997

COMMENT

One way in which these extracts illustrate that the debates on welfare futures are more complicated than that suggested by an approach which proposes a simple dichotomy between the state or the market, is the role each accords to the individual. For Green, as one might expect, the individual stands at the very heart of his argument. For Purdy too, though, the individual occupies a central place since it is to her or him that the Citizen's (or Basic) Income will be paid. However, this should not lead us to deny or underestimate the different place of the individual in their respective visions. Thus, whilst for Green the future welfare 'community' is peopled by a series of individuals unfettered by the debilitating demands of government, for Purdy the payment of a Citizen's Income is precisely the mechanism which ties the individual and government together. The individual is tied into a system of redistribution, or, as Purdy puts it, a tax-transfer system. Moreover, this system of taxation provides the ground for the creation of a framework of sentiments and a way of thinking – a structure of feeling. This makes it clear that the idea of self-reliance is the pivotal point of distinction between these two writers.

structure of feeling

This distinction becomes clearer when we contrast the role each accords the realm of 'the public'. Green makes it clear that in his vision 'the public' must have as minimal a role as possible – indeed, he sees public policies as impediments to individual enterprise and self-reliance. Thus, state agencies and monetary and fiscal policies must be limited to working for the enhancement of the individual's capacities in these tasks. In contrast, Purdy places the realm of 'the public' at the centre of his vision for the future; indeed, his Citizen's Income is one expression of this. In other respects, 'the public' would provide the mechanisms by which market-generated inequalities would be minimized, redistribution would be effected, and modes of connection between sections of 'the people' would be constituted. Beyond this, it is through 'the public' – understood as an 'active partnership between state and civil society' – that any excesses of the state and market would be curbed. It is this which enhances 'society's capacity to handle distributive conflict without recourse to either brute coercion or the impersonal discipline of the market'.

If the place of 'the public' occupies contrasting positions in these two extracts, that of 'the market' is more complex. One could be excused for assuming that in Green's vision the free operation of the market would be a sufficient condition for ensuring the kind of welfare 'community' he advocates. But he makes it clear that the market is only one element for ensuring individual initiative and responsibility. Alongside this, and perhaps of even greater importance, are the issues of a transformed morality and the disconnection between law and politics. For Green, morality and individual self-reliance and initiative are intimately connected since a moral society is precisely one in which individual self-reliance and individual service to others is the rule. Purdy is no less concerned with morality, but for him this would centre on a commitment to social justice (rather than voluntary service) and a sense of collective interest rather than narrow self- or sectional interest.

This is why, despite the differences between the two authors' positions, economic growth alone cannot provide the sufficient condition underpinning their visions of a welfare future. On its own, economic growth does not enter into and transform the wider political and cultural views and practices which are so central to any system of organizing the production and delivery of welfare services and benefits.

■ ■ ■

How do these two extracts illustrate the idea of a 'moral community' referred to at the beginning of section 1.1?

ACTIVITY 3.5(B)

Set 2 Reading for representations of the national popular

In the Introduction to this book it was pointed out that the restructuring of the social democratic welfare state involved more than just a set of overlapping reorganizations of systems for the production and delivery of welfare services and benefits. Certainly such restructuring was carried out (see **Hughes and Lewis, 1998**), but this was effected in a context in which the very meaning of the welfare state – what it stood for or represented – became subject to profound contestation. Central to this contestation was a struggle over how to imagine or construct the relationship between 'the people' and the nation-state. The idea of the national popular was utilized as one way of conceptualizing the struggle over how 'the people' were constituted. This idea was then elaborated in the introduction to this chapter so that the national popular was said to refer to:

■ a set of meanings about 'the nation' (and its people);

■ a field of legitimate political intervention;

■ sets of identifications across a range of social divisions.

With these points in mind, you should now re-read Extracts 3.5 and 3.6 and consider how each constructs a vision of the national popular. As you do so, it will be helpful to bear the following questions in mind:

1   Which, if any, social groupings or divisions are identified in the two extracts – for example, those of gender, 'race', (dis)ability, or divisions between (welfare) dependency or (welfare) independence?

2   What forms of material goods or services are envisioned as connecting diverse sections of 'the people' – for example, transfer payments, welfare benefits or services and tax systems?

3   What forms of symbolic connection between diverse sections of 'the people' are envisioned – for example, through senses of belonging or moral commitments to a wider 'community', and forms of voluntary activity?

4   To what extent is the field of welfare constructed as a legitimate site of state or public activity?

COMMENT

The first thing to note are the very different social groups and divisions referred to by the two authors. Green refers to the traditional two-parent family and the division between the 'dependent poor' and 'independent citizenship'. Purdy, in contrast, refers to the divisions of gender, class, 'race' and ethnicity as they affect the distribution of income, work and social power. The social categories to which each refers play a pivotal role in their respective arguments for the future shape of the welfare regime and are reflected further in the forms of material goods and services which they each propose as characteristic of their imagined futures. Thus, because Green foregrounds the divide between dependence and independence, and the traditional rather than other forms of family, he is concerned to emphasize the role that increased tax thresholds for individuals and married people, and child tax allowances, together with private care and voluntary association, will play in providing the connections between segments of 'the people'.

Similarly, we can see an integral connection between the social divisions highlighted by Purdy and the Citizen's Income he proposes. Thus, because he focuses on the ways in which certain social divisions affect the distribution of income, work and power, he is able to strengthen his argument for a Citizen's Income. This is because Citizen's Income is the mechanism through which to begin to overcome inequalities and through which to construct forms of material connection among unequal categories of the population. This, then, extends to the forms of symbolic connection which Purdy envisages – equality of status, active involvement in public affairs, social justice and the formation of moral communities which extend beyond market or sectional interests. For Green, these symbolic connections take the form of action for self-reliance, personal and familial responsibility, and involvement in voluntary activity. In promoting these forms of symbolic connection among members of a welfare community, Green suggests that he is simply arguing for a return to a past which was undermined by the emergence of the welfare state. As such, he invokes a vision of 'the past' in which forms of tradition are invented and through which the 'naturalness' or 'normality' of his vision can be constructed.

Finally, the extent to which the field of welfare is constructed as a legitimate site of state or public activity varies enormously in the two extracts. For Purdy, the legitimacy of such activity is central to his vision since it is the state which designs and implements the tax system which funds the Citizen's Income and through which a new 'structure of feeling' emerges. In addition, it is the state which promotes and facilitates public debate and involvement in the policy process. In direct contrast to this, Green sees such activity as legitimate only in so far as it promotes 'independence'. Thus state activity must be directed at the removal of obstacles which prevent the poor's endeavours for self-reliance, or at the promotion of labour mobility. The state (or government as he refers to it) must also take action for constitutional reform which separates law and politics. Beyond this the state should do no more than ensure the existence of a residual welfare regime.

From a distinctive position on the right of the political spectrum, Green, then, is arguing for a new vision of the relation between the individual, the community and the state in which the central organizing principle is a system of *morals* which privileges the individual and the private. This morality is the nexus around which 'community' is formed and which guides the establishment and operation of the system of welfare (see also, for example, Chapter 2, section 3). Purdy's alternative vision of a welfare regime is one in which a notion of 'the public' provides the central connective tissue between the individual, the state and welfare. This is also a moral vision about the possible shape that a welfare regime in the UK may take in the twenty-first century, for, as he notes, not only have proposals for the reform of the welfare state come from both Right and Left, but also the classification of welfare states into types is about 'the values, assumptions, commitments and institutions which, taken together, determine the character of that state's *social policy regime*' (Purdy, 1994, p.32).

■ ■ ■

6   The persistence of inequalities

In this section I want to focus on the links between, on the one hand, the form of citizenship which was delineated by Marshall and which characterized the social democratic welfare state, and, on the other hand, the issue of inequalities produced through social divisions of gender. The implications of the demands for an expanded notion of rights and entitlements which have been expressed by feminist groups, gay and lesbian groups, black groups, and disabled peoples' groups suggest that to retain the idea of class as the only or main element in a politics of citizenship is limited and fails to recognize a whole range of fragmented and diversified social relations. The inequalities which attach to divisions of gender, 'race'/ethnicity and able-bodiedness produce categories of belonging which cut across and expand the idea of citizenship. They raise fundamental issues about the social subject equated to that of the citizen in Marshall (1996). As **Hughes (1998)** has pointed out, this figure was the white, male breadwinner whose citizenship rights were expressed, as much as anything, as a right and duty to earn a family wage. Moreover, the system of welfare which developed after the Second World War in the UK was centred on this idea of a family wage, with all the dependencies within the family which resulted from it.

male breadwinner

family wage

To gain an understanding of how the dominant notion of citizenship which prevailed in the social democratic welfare state constructed forms of gendered dependency we need to return to the terrain laid out by Marshall. Extract 3.7, taken from an article by Gillian Pascall, allows us to do this by illustrating a feminist critique of this form of citizenship. Importantly, it enables us to draw out the difference between formal political equality and substantive inequality in all three elements of citizenship identified by Marshall. These inequalities

Expanded citizenship?

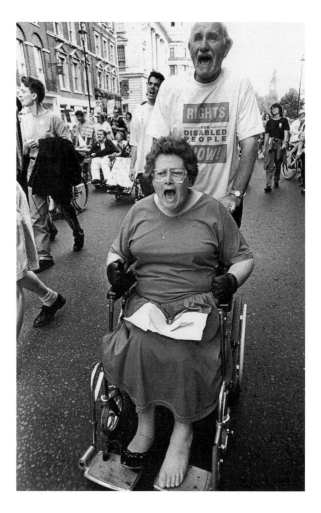

derive from the differential and subordinated position of women in the actually existing social relations of welfare. It focuses on the ways in which the divide between the public and the private constitutes the materiality of gendered inequalities in citizenship. As you read through it, you should note the limitations on women's citizenship rights and the ways in which the traditional family produces women's dependency and subordinated citizenship.

Extract 3.7 Pascall: 'Limits to citizenship – women and the family'

Marshall's classic analysis of … the relationship between citizenship and social class was not matched by questioning about citizenship and dependency in the family (Pascall, 1986). My concern … is with analysing ways in which women's citizenship in practice is restricted by family dependency …

Feminist debates have made the question of the relationship between the family and citizenship as fundamental and problematic as that between class and citizenship. …

In locating my argument here I start from the assumption that the division between public and private is problematic, as is women's customary location within the family.

Civil rights

It is usually assumed that civil rights are more firmly entrenched than social rights. There have been substantial gains in women's legal rights to person and property, but crucial areas of feminist writing concern the denial of such rights in practice: domestic violence and marital rape, relationships of dependency within marriage, and the 'compulsory altruism' of 'community care' may all be seen as aspects of the denial of women's civil rights. …

… women's increased access to employment has slackened the economic bonds of marriage and cohabitation for many women, loosening the knot between economic security and wifely duty. But women's relatively lower incomes and security from paid work still make women dependent on the men with whom they live; and British social surveys indicate that wifely duties have a reducing hold on peoples' ideals, but are alive and well in practice.

Economic dependence is increased by the physical and emotional dependence of others – of children and elderly relatives. While housewifery as a primary economic role has gone into decline for younger women with access to jobs, policies for 'community care' put pressure on a mainly older and mainly female population to do unpaid caring work. …

Another aspect of civil rights is raised by the extreme needs of some dependent relatives and the isolation and consequent loss of autonomy of those who care for them. Civil liberty may be at stake in the more severe situations, and again there is an issue of state neglect in providing appropriate alternatives. …

All these examples call into question the extent of women's civil rights and citizenship within the family. Power and privacy in marriage relationships, economic dependency and its link with unpaid work roles, and the 'compulsory altruism' of community care are aspects of family relationships which limit women's civil rights. …

Social rights

There is no shortage of evidence about women's unequal position in relation to rights derived from the market and rights derived from social welfare policies (Lister, 1990a,b) This section will focus on a topic which has special significance for the public/private boundary – social security rights connected with paid and unpaid work.

The attachment of social rights to paid employment is a significant basis for the recognition of citizens in practice. Beveridge ensured that paid employment was a key basis for citizenship in Britain with his scheme for social insurance: it was elaborated from the notion that the needs to be met were those arising from a break in men's employment, and that the mechanism should be compulsory contributions while in employment. His clarity about women's work and position in marriage did not lead him to recommend benefits accruing directly in relation to unpaid work: but rather to a very uncitizen-like dependence on their husbands. …

… By attaching social security to paid employment, national insurance still penalizes women for carrying out their 'vital work' [that is, unpaid domestic labour].

There are some policies in which women's unpaid work is acknowledged as entitling them to social rights: credits for family responsibility (counting towards national insurance), and child benefit (paid to women on behalf of their children) are two British ones. But such benefits are lower in practice than the rights accruing as a result of paid work – rights to flat-rate pensions rather than graduated ones, to benefit for one's children but not for oneself.

The Invalid Care Allowance [ICA] is an interesting British example of a social benefit relating to unpaid work – entitlement depends on giving up paid work to care for others. In some respects it belongs to notions of citizenship. Entitlement is based on the existence of caring needs, not on a contract to carry them out; there is no contract of duties, no procedure to control their enforcement. But ICA is also a critical case for measuring the extent of citizenship rights deriving from unpaid work. At first it was not available to married women on the twin assumptions of natural duty and dependence on husbands ... Now – thanks to [a] ruling by the European Court – married women may claim ... ICA is becoming a significant social security benefit for women, who constitute 86 per cent of beneficiaries. But its level was originally set at 60 per cent of the level of contributory benefits. The deliberate intention was to privilege contributory benefits over non-contributory ones ... Citizenship derived from paid employment is thus better than citizenship derived through unpaid work. ...

Duties

The assumption of paid work as the central citizenship obligation underpins many debates – about workfare, training, the conditionality of benefits (Plant, 1988, pp.14–15). Certain social rights have followed market rights in being tied to paid work, sometimes becoming a means of enforcement.

But women's access to well-paid work is much less than men's; concomitantly their obligations to do unpaid work are greater. The impact of childcare on women's ability to do paid work and to contribute towards benefits has long been acknowledged. ...

But who enforces the duty to unpaid work (Taylor-Gooby, 1991)? In the case of paid work great attention is paid to questions of incentives, so that social benefits do not bring the same rewards as market benefits.

Obligations to unpaid work are not socially policed or materially rewarded. Cultural and economic pressures may suffice to ensure that women do their duty. ... [Some writers] have speculated about whether we can rescue the concept of citizenship by finding ways to spread the obligation for unpaid work (Jordan, 1991; Taylor-Gooby, 1991). While I like the objective, I remain sceptical about the means to this end. Neither commodification of the domestic world – with market incentives applied to caring work – nor 'compulsory altruism' (Land and Rose, 1985) applied this time to men are particularly attractive alternatives. ...

Despite [this] reconceptualizing citizenship to acknowledge gender-specific social roles – without entrenching them – is the more inviting prospect.

References

Jordan, B. (1991) 'Efficiency, justice and the obligations of citizenship: the basic income approach', paper presented to Anglo-German Social Policy Conference, Nottingham.

Land, H. and Rose, H. (1985) 'Compulsory altruism for some, or an altruistic society for all', in Bean, P., Ferris, J. and Whynes, D. (eds) *In Defence of Welfare*, London, Tavistock.

Lister, R. (1990a) 'Women, economic dependency and citizenship', *Journal of Social Policy*, vol.19, no.4, pp.445–67.

Lister, R. (1990b) *The Exclusive Society: Citizenship and the Poor*, London, Child Poverty Action Group.

Pascall, G. (1986) *Social Policy: A Feminist Analysis*, London, Tavistock.

Plant, R. (1988) *Citizenship, Rights and Socialism*, London, Fabian Society (Fabian Tracts; 531).

Taylor-Gooby, P. (1991) 'Scrounging, moral hazard and unwaged work: citizenship and human need', paper presented at Social Policy Association Conference, University of Nottingham.

(Pascall, 1993, pp.113–14, 116–22, 125)

In this extract, Pascall notes the advances in women's material position (via access to paid employment); their legal position (for example, in the right to hold property in their own right); and their symbolic position (expressed in, for example, a decrease in the notion of 'wifely duty'). However, her emphasis is on the ways in which women still occupy a second-class or subordinated citizenship status. This subordinated status is a result of the sexual division of labour within the family and household and especially because of the unequal responsibility for caring which women have.

To what extent do you think that Green would see this kind of dependency as indicative of a serious problem within the welfare regime?

Such caring responsibilities are social labours but are not recognized or valued as such. Pascall argues that this is demonstrated by the lack of publicly provided alternatives for unpaid caring. Moreover, the assumption that women will carry out caring responsibilities was woven into the fabric of the social democratic welfare state as evidenced by the idea of the male breadwinner and the family wage. Thus the male insurance contribution established the framework which ensured women's lack of full citizenship rights. The central argument made by Pascall is that the social and symbolic division between paid and unpaid work reflects and reproduces women's subordinate status in the citizenship stakes. Pascall, then, draws our attention to the ways in which the 'citizen' has been constituted around a male norm and a traditional family, thus allowing us to see that citizenship itself has been constructed in and through the institution of gender.

6.1 Moving beyond gender inequality

If the 'gender effect' has had a profound impact on the substantive operation of citizenship, particularly in relation to welfare benefits and services, the question remains as to how to imagine things being different. Nancy Fraser is a North American feminist who has considered the question of how to construct a welfare regime and welfare subject in a way which overcomes and surpasses these gendered inequalities. Starting from a critique of actually existing welfare relations, Fraser attempts to construct a way of imagining the future relations of welfare which has the pursuit of gender equality at its heart. Extract 3.8 reproduces some of what she proposes, but before reading this it is vitally important to be aware of three points in particular. First, it should be remembered that Fraser is offering an *ideal-typical* model of the future structure of welfare relations. This model is built around an act of imagination because she postulates 'contrary to fact, a world in which … [her model is] feasible in that … [the] economic and political preconditions are in place' (Fraser, 1997, pp.43–4). Despite the model's imaginative status (indeed because of it), it provides an opportunity for thinking explicitly about the implications for the distribution of symbolic and material resources if the figure of the citizen is constructed around a new imagery. This is the second point to bear in mind. The third point is that Fraser conceives of gender equality (and its pursuit) as a complex idea and *process* comprising seven elements or normative principles, each of which would need to be fulfilled if gender equality were to be achieved in the new system of welfare relations. The seven principles are:

1   anti-poverty

2   anti-exploitation

3 income equality

4 leisure-time equality

5 equality of respect

6 anti-marginalization

7 anti-androcentrism.

To what extent do you think these seven principles correspond to the gender inequalities identified by Pascall?

Each of these seven elements are currently axes of *inequality* between men and women, rooted, in large part, in the structures which act as the conduits for the distribution of symbolic and material resources, including those associated with welfare. With these principles in mind, Fraser attempts to devise a model of welfare which will both reconstruct the 'citizen' around a new social figure and have the outcome of producing the most gender parity in domestic, waged and civic life. Extract 3.8 outlines Fraser's model.

ACTIVITY 3.6

Read through Extract 3.8 and, as you do so, make a note of the following:

■ which subject is at the centre of the model;

■ the elements of the current sexual division of labour that the model is aimed at destabilizing;

■ how Fraser's model envisages the relation between public institutions and private households;

■ the implications for the split between the public and the private.

Extract 3.8 Imaginative act 3. Fraser: 'The universal caregiver'

The key to achieving gender equity in a postindustrial welfare state, then, is to make women's current life-patterns the norm for everyone. Women today often combine breadwinning and caregiving, albeit with great difficulty and strain. A postindustrial welfare state must ensure that men do the same, while redesigning institutions so as to eliminate the difficulty and strain. We might call this vision *Universal Caregiver*.

What, then, might such a welfare state look like? Unlike Caregiver Parity, its employment sector would not be divided into two different tracks; all jobs would be designed for workers who are caregivers, too ... Unlike Universal Breadwinner, however, employees would not be assumed to shift all carework to social services. Some informal carework would be publicly supported and integrated on a par with paid work in a single social-insurance system. Some would be performed in households by relatives and friends, but such households would not necessarily be heterosexual nuclear families. Other supported carework would be located outside households altogether – in civil society. In state-funded but locally organized institutions, childless adults, older people, and others without kin-based responsibilities would join parents and others in democratic, self-managed carework activities.

A Universal Caregiver welfare state would promote gender equity by effectively dismantling the gendered opposition between breadwinning and caregiving. It would integrate activities that are currently separated from one another, eliminate their gender-coding, and encourage men to perform them too. This, however, is tantamount to a wholesale restructuring of the institution of gender. ... By deconstructing the opposition between breadwinning and caregiving, moreover, Universal Caregiver would simultaneously deconstruct the associated opposition between bureaucratized public institutional settings and intimate private domestic settings. Treating civil society as an additional site for carework, ... Universal Caregiver promises expansive new possibilities for enriching the substance of social life and for promoting equal participation.

Only by embracing the Universal Caregiver vision, moreover, can we mitigate potential conflicts among our seven component principles of gender equity and minimize the need for trade-offs. ... *Achieving gender equity in a postindustrial welfare state, then, requires deconstructing gender.* ...

The trick is to imagine a social world in which citizens' lives integrate wage earning, caregiving, community activism, political participation, and involvement in the associational life of civil society – while also leaving time for some fun.

(Fraser, 1997, pp.61–2)

COMMENT

It is clear that the subject at the heart of this model is what Fraser calls the 'Universal Caregiver'. It is from the occupation of this subject position that citizenship rights and responsibilities flow. Moreover, this model constructs *all* adults as equally caregivers and wage earners regardless of their sex. In this way, the model seeks to destabilize the existing division of labour between women and men, in which women are constructed as, and indeed are responsible for, most carework, and men are constructed as the primary wage earners. Such a destabilization could only be achieved by a reorganization of labour markets, but it would also require a radical reorganization of carework. Central to this would be a redistribution of carework to numerous sites – publicly funded institutions, diverse types of household and smaller, locally controlled units. Importantly, all adults would become responsible for carework. Similarly, this redistribution to numerous sites and all adults would be part of a process whereby caring was accorded equal *symbolic* value with wage-earning. The overall result of these changes would be a wholesale dismantling of the current system of gender relations and, with it, the split between the public and the private, which is one expression of this system.

This example illustrates how feminism as a political strategy and vision enables a reformulation of the issue of citizenship. By focusing on the gender inequalities inherent within the liberal version of citizenship, particularly as it was expressed in the social democratic welfare state, feminists have been able to (a) challenge the universal and unitary subject of welfare embodied in the Beveridgean welfare state; and (b) question what will be, and who will decide, the terms of inclusion in the welfare community. Moreover, despite some similarities with arguments for basic income such as that proposed by Purdy (see also Gorz, 1992; Jordan, 1992), Fraser's vision has a wider remit. Whilst all those who support a form of basic income share a commitment to a form of citizenship which would promote an increased freedom from paid labour, Fraser is self-consciously attempting to imagine a system in which freedom from *unpaid* labour is a direct objective, and not simply a by-product of a redistribution of paid labour. The redistribution of leisure time and symbolic value is also central to Fraser's feminist future.

■ ■ ■

'Universal Caregiver'

Limited citizenship: children – duties not rights

---

2. The following Code of Behaviour was established and agreed by all staff and children

Highgate Primary School
Code of Behaviour

1. Please move quietly and sensibly around the school.

2. No bullying, name calling, fighting, rough behaviour or "play fighting".
Please don't get involved.

3. Please be kind, helpful, polite and respectful of others and try to be a good listener.

4. Please look after our school and the equipment and keep the classrooms tidy.

5. Please work well, stay on task and do your best.

6. Never throw things – you might hurt someone.

****

BE FRIENDLY
Make someone happy every day!

ACTIVITY 3.7

Before going on to the next section, take some time to fill in the following grid in which you compare and contrast the main elements of the three 'imaginative acts'.

Comparing and contrasting the 'imaginative acts'

	Green	Purdy	Fraser
Issues to be addressed			
Main objectives to be achieved			
Means by which to achieve objectives			
Forms of material and symbolic ties connecting 'the people'			

7   The borders of citizenship

In each of the preceding sections we have considered the inequalities which ensued from the construction of a normative figure at the heart of the idea of citizenship. Thus we have seen how, despite formal equality of status, the Marshallian idea of making distinctions between types of service within the welfare state led to inequalities of class and disability. We have also seen how the construction of a male breadwinner as the citizen resulted in inequalities organized around gender difference. In considering these inequalities and the subordinated inclusions and exclusions which actually or potentially result from the construction of citizenship in this way, we have, however, kept the focus of our discussion on citizenship relations *within* the nation-state. At first sight this may seem inevitable given that the rights and duties of citizenship are granted and protected by a specific nation-state. In this sense, then, citizenship is a profoundly national issue since it organizes the respective rights and responsibilities between the individual and the nation-state. However, in this section I want to expand the parameters of our discussion and think about some of the issues which arise when we extend our focus beyond the borders of the nation-state. Yuval-Davis (1997) has succinctly summed up the issues:

> Citizenship needs to be examined, not just in terms of the state, but often in relation to multiple formal and informal citizenships in more than one country. Most importantly, these citizenships need to be viewed from a perspective which would include the different positioning of the different states as well as the different positionings of individuals and groupings within states.
>
> (Yuval-Davis, 1997, p.75)

This short quotation raises a wide number of issues which I want to consider here in relation to the UK's history as an *imperial* nation-state, and the more recent challenges raised by the emergence of the European Union and the UK's membership of it. Taking these issues as the point of departure for our discussion, I want to consider the following:

■   the relationship between citizenship and nationality in terms of the evolution of legal definitions of British citizenship in the twentieth century;

■   the extent to which the emergence of a form of supra-national state – in the shape of the EU – opens a space to renegotiate citizenship rights in a way which allows for a greater degree of inclusivity.

7.1   The imperial citizen: the evolution of an uneasy partnership

If the 1940s were the moment when the welfare state was being brought into being, the Labour government of the time was also turning its attention to the development of a legal definition of British nationality and citizenship. Despite this and later attempts to define and clarify the meaning of British citizenship, the discursive connections between nationality, national identity and citizenship have developed in the absence of any written constitution which clearly establishes the criteria by which citizenship status is accorded and, indeed, defended. So, while the category 'British Citizen' did not exist in law until 1981 (Dummett, 1994, p.75), it is within the interplay of 'nationality' and 'national identity' that the rights and duties of British 'citizenship' have expanded and narrowed at different points in time (Cesarani, 1996, p.67). How can we explain this paradox? One way into grasping the shifts and paradoxes which have characterized nationality, national identity and citizenship within the UK is to look at the development of immigration and nationality law over the twentieth century. This will enable us to see the ways in which the boundaries of the nation have been drawn and redrawn over the decades of the twentieth century and, with them, the constructions of who 'the people' are.

In legal terms the definition of what it meant, and who could have British nationality and citizenship, must be understood as a thoroughly imperial development linked to the rise (and fall) of the British Empire in the nineteenth and twentieth centuries. In this sense, British citizenship is coterminous with the development of social rights as defined by Marshall in his evolutionary schema. However, in order to grasp the confusion and opacity of what is meant by British nationality or citizenship, it is necessary to begin our thinking much further back than this and at least to feudal times – a point already signalled by the term and status 'British subject'. From the thirteenth to the twentieth century this was the name given to ever wider sections of the population of the British Isles, as the state which today is the United Kingdom progressively came into being. 'Britons' were not citizens, they were subjects of the crown, a crown who was sovereign and to whom one owed allegiance. Birthplace (or *ius soli*) was what determined this status and the national belonging which accompanied it. One's exact social position within the status of British subjecthood was linked to the ownership and non-ownership of land, but the predominant feature was birth within the boundaries of the crown's jurisdiction. The development of an established, Protestant church, and the emergence of parliamentary dominance over the monarchy, meant that subjecthood was redefined to include a confessional and democratic dimension (Colley, 1992; Cesarani, 1996, p.58). However, these only modified the category and status of subjecthood rather than leading to its demise or replacement by that of 'citizen'. As such, the people of the UK were defined as British subjects, with the joint sovereignty of the crown and parliament the symbol of the nation and central to the constructed national identity.

These developments occurred within the context of a continually expanding state expressed by the metamorphosis of England into England and Wales; into Britain; into the United Kingdom – a nation-state achieved by the Act of Union of 1801 with Ireland, and modified in 1922 with the division of the island of Ireland into Eire and Northern Ireland. It is also worth noting that, up until the civil rights movement in the late 1960s, the right to vote in Northern Ireland remained tied to ownership of property and householder status. In addition to this, Britain rose to an unprecedented position of imperial dominance, so that British subjecthood was not confined only to inhabitants of the British Isles. Thus, all those born within the ('white') dominions, such as Canada, Australia and South Africa, and within the colonies, such as those in West Africa, the Caribbean and South Asia, were also British subjects. Moreover, all those who had the status of 'British subject' were formally equal, in a similar way to the formal equality accorded citizens born and residing within the British state. This was, then, an *imperial* nationality and category of political belonging and it is in the context of the unravelling of empire that the forms of British citizenship which have emerged since the 1940s are to be understood.

Accompanying this imperial nationality was the formation of a national identity. From our discussion so far we can identify at least two elements which formed the central strands of this national identity:

1   birth within one of the lands which were part of the domain of the crown;

2   Protestantism, especially, though not exclusively, Anglicanism.

That these criteria formed the boundaries of the national identity had two effects which are relevant to the concerns of this book. On the one hand, it was against these that the category of 'alien' was constructed. On the other hand, it was precisely around these criteria as the foundations of the national identity that the tensions produced by the construction of a formal equality among all holding the imperial nationality clustered. The links between the construction of national identity and the construction of the 'alien' are potently illustrated by the fevered debate about the implications of Jewish immigration from Eastern Europe from the 1880s through to first years of the twentieth century. As Cesarani (1996, p.60) has pointed out, the tensions and instabilities of national identity are often most starkly exposed by the presence of immigrants, especially if these immigrants are constructed as the 'alien', as was the case with these Jewish migrants. Thus, just as 'coloured immigrants' in the 1960s and 1970s, and the Muslim presence in the 1980s and 1990s, acutely posed questions of national belonging and citizenship (see, for example, discussion of the Muslim schools debate in **Lewis, 1998b**; also Dwyer, 1993; Miller, 1995), so too did the Jewish presence at the turn of the nineteenth and twentieth centuries. What this illustrates is the ways in which religion (Judaism or Islam, in this case) or skin colour can become the sign of the 'alien' and it was this form of symbolic process which provided the background to the 1905 Aliens Act. In this context, then, the construction of the category 'alien' is as much about the construction of a *cultural* category of belonging as it is about the construction of a *legal* category – defining who has a right of entry to the country or that of access to welfare goods and services. Indeed, the same can be said about the immigration legislation passed since the 1960s.

If the 1905 Aliens Act marked a highwater moment in the distinction between 'British subject' and 'alien', the internal tensions contained within the category 'British subject' were to reach boiling point in the decades up to the 1948 British Nationality Act. At several points during this time the universal principle central to the imperial nationality was reaffirmed. For example, the 1914 British Nationality and Status of Aliens Act had confirmed that the principle of *ius soli* (nationality by birthright) extended to all born within the province of the British crown's realm, and this was reiterated at the Imperial Conference held in the 1930s (Paul, 1997).

Despite these frequent reaffirmations of a universal and equal status and nationality across the whole empire/commonwealth, the governments of some territories began to express increasing resistance to it. Canada played a pivotal role in this in both the 1930s and 1940s (Paul, 1997; Dummett, 1994), though in the earlier case they dropped their proposal to create an independent Canadian nationality and citizenship. However, in 1945 Canada again proposed a bill which would break the principle of an imperial nationality and establish 'Canadian citizenship [as] the primary nationality and making British subjecthood a secondary status' (Paul, 1997, p.14). Two years later, India too – and, upon partition, India and Pakistan – announced plans for their own, independent nationality and citizenship which would contest the imperial nationality as the primary one. It was in the face of these contestations to a universal British subjecthood that the 1948 British Nationality Act was passed, the main terms of which are listed in Table 3.1.

Table 3.1 Development of principal British Aliens, Nationality and Immigration Acts in the twentieth century

1905 Aliens Act	This was implemented in response to Jewish refugee migration from Eastern Europe. It established an immigration control bureau with the power of expulsion. It also contained a financial assets clause
1914 Aliens Restriction Act	This established Home Office control over the internal movement of those defined as 'aliens'. Also aliens now required to register with the police. Represented first radical shift in the prior right of aliens to free entry and movement unless specifically excluded
1914 British Nationality and Status of Aliens Act	This affirmed that all inhabitants of the UK, the dominions and the colonies were 'British subjects' owing allegiance to the crown. Did not allow for freedom of movement by all such inhabitants to all parts of the empire, but standardized naturalization procedures across the empire. Women were denied the ability to transmit British nationality to children; they also lost this nationality on marriage to an 'alien' man; but British men transmitted their nationality if married to an 'alien' woman
1919 Aliens Restriction (Amendment) Act	This continued the terms of the 1914 Aliens Act to peacetime. Removed right of former 'enemy aliens' to sit on juries or work for the government even if naturalized. If not naturalized, industrial or political 'subversion' could lead to deportation
1948 British Nationality Act	This established two main categories of citizenship: (i) citizens of the United Kingdom and Colonies (UKC); (ii) citizens of Commonwealth countries. Both of these had the imperial status of 'British subject' with the entitlement to settle in the UK. It equalled a political compromise which enabled retention of the imperial nationality whilst allowing for independent national citizenships. There was also a third category for citizens of Eire – who were deemed neither aliens nor subjects but had all the rights and duties of UKC subjects. Some have argued that this compromise resulted from the need for labour in Britain and the difficulties of policing the border between Northern Ireland and Eire (see Hickman, 1998)
1957 British Nationality Act	This allowed people defined as of 'pure European descent', despite neither themselves nor their fathers being born in the UK, to register as UKC citizens within five years
1962 Commonwealth Immigrants Act	This represented the first major modification in the rights of entry which attached to imperial nationality. Applicable only to those UKC subjects not born in the UK and not holding a British passport, it introduced a three-tiered work voucher system for would-be Commonwealth migrants. They could also enter for the purposes of study. The work voucher system was modified further in 1965
1968 Commonwealth Immigrants Act	This was passed in response to the 'Africanization' process in Kenya and in the context of a formal right of entry for UKC subjects. The Act denied automatic right of entry and settlement to those defined as 'Kenyan Asians'. Entry of UKC subjects was now only possible if they, or a parent or grandparent, were born, adopted, registered or naturalized in the UK. This situation contrasted to that of Kenyans of European descent who had had their right of entry protected in a special Nationality Act passed in 1964

1971 Immigration Act	This took the 'patriality' notion – that is, the ability to trace a connection to the UK through a grand/parent being born, naturalized, adopted or registered in the UK – to its logical conclusion by restricting British nationality to patrials only. All those who held UKC citizenship/nationality but were born in the Commonwealth and had no grand/parental link to the UK were, henceforth, deprived of UKC rights of entry and settlement. Non-patrials, as these people were now called, were effectively treated the same as aliens. Irish citizens remained free from immigration control if they entered via the UK, Ireland or the Channel Islands – known as the Common Travel Area. Since 1974, however, they have been liable to control of their freedom of movement via the Prevention of Terrorism Act
1981 British Nationality Act	This represented the end of the principle of *ius soli*. From 1986 onwards, citizenship would only be accorded to UK born or naturalized people and their UK born or naturalized children. Three categories of citizenship were established: (i) British citizenship; (ii) British Dependent Territories citizenship; (iii) British Overseas citizenship. The Act also established that those children born in the UK but to parents who are not legally settled here would only be eligible for citizenship after 10 years continuous residence
1988 Immigration Act	This removed the right of certain British citizens to be joined in the UK by their spouse, making worse an already tortuous and bureaucratic process for dealing with applications for family reunification

Sources: Commission for Racial Equality, 1985; Dummett, 1994; Cesarani, 1996; Guild, 1996; Paul, 1997

This brief history enables us to establish four key points. These are that:

1   Citizenship is about sets of relationships *within* a nation-state.

2   It is about the establishment of the boundaries of the nation-state against which 'aliens' are defined – that is, the boundaries of one nation-state against others.

3   In the case of the UK at least, citizenship must also be seen as emerging within the context of a state whose power and authority extended far beyond its geographical boundaries and was, therefore, a supra-national state.

4   Citizenship is about constructing constituencies of national belonging as well as rights and duties to be exercised in relation to the state.

To the extent that nationality and immigration law construct constituencies of belonging, these are *cultural* processes and artefacts. This is so because they constantly produce and remake images or representations of 'the people' (and therefore 'the alien'). However, the degree to which laws of nationality and immigration actually facilitate a broadly *inclusive* understanding of national belonging is open to contestation. This is clear from Extracts 3.9 and 3.10.

AN IMPORTANT ANNOUNCEMENT ON BEHALF OF THE COUNCIL OF THE CITY OF LEICESTER, ENGLAND

The City Council of Leicester, England, believe that many families in Uganda are considering moving to Leicester.
If YOU are thinking of doing so it is very important you should know that PRESENT CONDITIONS IN THE CITY ARE VERY DIFFERENT FROM THOSE MET BY EARLIER SETTLERS. They are:–

HOUSING – several thousands of families are already on the Council's waiting list.

EDUCATION – hundreds of children are awaiting places in schools

SOCIAL AND HEALTH SERVICES – already stretched to the limit

IN YOUR OWN INTERESTS AND THOSE OF YOUR FAMILY YOU SHOULD ACCEPT THE ADVICE OF THE UGANDA RESETTLEMENT BOARD AND NOT COME TO LEICESTER

NURSES FOR BRITAIN

QUALIFIED AND SEMI-QUALIFIED NURSES ARE URGENTLY REQUIRED FOR HOSPITALS AND HOMES AT TOP AGENCY RATES
SOME RESIDENCY AVAILABLE

WRITE IMMEDIATELY FOR APPLICATION FORM AND FURTHER DETAILS
OUR SERVICE IS FREE OF ANY CHARGE OR COMMISSION

RELIANCE SERVICES NURSES AGENCY

49 Great Ormond Street
LONDON W.C.1.
Telephone: 01 405 9038

Imperial citizenship: legacies and paradoxes (two advertisements from page 2 of the Uganda Argus, *6 October 1972)*

ACTIVITY 3.8

You should now read Extracts 3.9 and 3.10 which are taken from the work of Ann Dummett and Kathleen Paul respectively. As you read, make a note of the following:

■ how each author characterizes the emergence of nationality law since 1948;

■ what the authors say were the effects of nationality and immigration law on different constituencies of people;

■ the extent to which each extract suggests that British nationality law constructed an inclusive category of national belonging.

Extract 3.9 Dummett: 'Chaos and inclusion'

In 1948 a British Nationality Act was passed at Westminster which retained the name of subject for citizens of all Commonwealth countries, including the United Kingdom and its colonies, but which established a new citizenship of the United Kingdom and Colonies alongside new, independent citizenships that the self-governing British Dominions were creating, first in Canada, then in India and elsewhere. This citizenship had no rights attached to it; one had rights as a subject still because [this] status of subject was retained alongside the new citizenship. ...

Since 1962 we have had a series of Immigration Acts which have taken away the right of large numbers of people to enter and stay in the United Kingdom, and the restrictions have been, not in terms but in effect, racially discriminatory. ... Most countries define their citizenship, assume that citizens have right of residence, and then devise immigration control systems for aliens. Britain decides whom to allow in, out of her existing nationals as well as aliens, and then defines her citizenship accordingly. ...

Our system is an almost unbelievable muddle ... However, there are some virtues in it, mainly the creation of historical accident rather than of principle or policy, and these are well worth considering. ...

British nationality has always been acquired primarily by the rule of birthplace or *ius soli* – simply because that was the feudal rule in the thirteenth century for making a person a subject of the king. The principle was, unfortunately, slightly modified in 1981 but remains the main rule. This has meant that Britain which, contrary to popular belief has always been a country of immigration, has absorbed a large variety of people without difficulty, the British-born children of immigrants having been fully and undoubtedly British and regarded as such. ... Our whole national history and character would undoubtedly have been different without the twin effects of *ius soli* and continual immigration from outside. We have been, one might say, a multicultural society without knowing it, so unselfconscious has this absorption been. We have not been free of xenophobia: there have been many ugly outbreaks of hostility to foreigners at different times. And yet absorption has been possible, strangely enough, without there being any demand until very recently for immigrants to conform to our ways.

(Dummett, 1994, pp.77–9)

Extract 3.10 Paul: 'Imperial compromise: national exclusion'

... the politics of citizenship was not the result of confusion but rather reflected competing communities of 'Britishness' which challenged the policy-making elites' presentation of a single and singular British imperial national identity. Proclaiming equality as the universal nationality policy enabled policy makers to propagate the image of the British Empire as a liberal, civilizing institution. In reality, this facade of equality was fractured along several lines ... [among them] ... the inequalities caused by the significance accorded skin color, ... it was this significance that had the most direct and immediate effect on concepts of British nationality.

The understanding of the world's population which made skin color the definitive signifier of group and national identity resulted in different communities of Britishness which reflected separate spheres of nationality. 'Racialization' created a fundamental contradiction between an inclusive legal nationality policy – the formal definition of who had the right to enter the country – and an exclusive constructed national identity – the informal notion of who really did or could belong. Thus, despite an imperial nationality and the facade of equality, the policy-making elite perceived emigrating UK residents, immigrating continental and Irish aliens, and migrating subjects of color as belonging to different communities of Britishness. As a result, each group experienced Britishness in a different way, their access to material wealth, education, and privilege conditioned by where they were perceived to 'fit' within the hierarchy of Britishness.

(Paul, 1997, p.xii)

COMMENT

The contrast between these two authors' characterization of the emergence of nationality law since 1948 is immediately clear. Whereas Dummett suggests that the confusion in the system is a result of 'historical accident' rather than 'principle or policy', Paul suggests quite the opposite. For her, the absence of such accident or 'confusion' points in the direction of political compromise – it was conscious policy but one which was driven by the presumed need to make the best out of the challenges posed to the imperial nationality which had hitherto been the status quo.

Importantly, this need for compromise was itself the product of the *de facto* inequalities of the imperial nationality expressed by the existence of what Paul calls 'competing communities of "Britishness"'. Central to this construction of differentiated categories of 'Britishness' is skin colour and a discourse of population which categorizes diverse peoples into 'races'. From this Paul argues that British

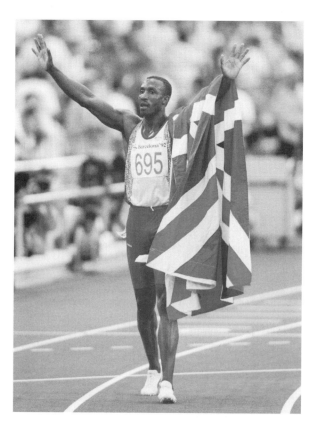

The iconic post-imperial Briton?

nationality was an *exclusive* category, organized around a hierarchy of actual or potential national belonging. This hierarchical categorization then affected the relative citizenship rights of each group, which she identifies as emigrating UK residents; incoming European and Irish migrants; and incoming migrants from the Caribbean, South Asia and Africa. Each of these groups had a greater or lesser chance of being included as 'true' members of the British national community – as being of 'the people'.

Despite the recognition that immigration law has been 'racially discriminatory' in effect, Dummett 'reads' the constitutive effects of the legislation in a different way. Thus, for her, the overall thrust of British nationality and immigration law has been towards *inclusion*. This is so despite some incidences of xenophobia and despite the fact that she recognizes that some who have been defined as nationals are denied automatic right of entry.

■ ■ ■

The contrasts between these two 'readings' of the effects of British nationality and immigration law can, in part, be explained by the authors' different interpretative starting-points. Thus Paul makes what we can call a 'cultural' reading, alongside a legal/empirical one, which is evidenced by her concern to elicit and highlight the ways in which these laws reflected and constructed particular images of who belonged to the British nation. To put it another way, she is concerned with the processes of *representation* by which national belonging and identity are produced. Dummett, on the other hand, focuses more on the empirical and legal aspects alone – who is allowed in, on what criteria, and what actions have occurred against those coming in. She is not really concerned to analyse representations. Despite this, her own analysis constructs a particular image of British nationality and immigration law. Thus, in Dummett's characterization, Britain is represented as an *inclusive* society, whilst for Paul, it is represented as an *exclusive* society. For our purposes what matters is the construction of who can be British and on what terms. The empirical detail of numbers of emigrants and immigrants is only of interest in terms of the role they play in the construction of competing representations of 'the people' and national belonging.

7.2 The redirected gaze: citizenship in the context of the European Union

If the 1980s marked the culmination of the process by which the meaning and scope of British citizenship and nationality were increasingly narrowed, the 1990s marked the moment when the thorny questions of national belonging and identity were once again sharply posed. Two factors can be identified as symbolic of this reworking of 'old' questions. First, the coming into force of the Maastricht Treaty in November 1993 and, second, the beginnings of processes of devolution within the UK in 1997. In relation to the European Union there are two issues which I want to explore briefly. These are:

1   the rights and duties associated with the emergence of citizenship of the EU;

2   the extent to which such a citizenship marks the beginnings of a separation between nationality and citizenship rights.

The question of devolution within the UK raises a number of profound constitutional, political and cultural issues, but here I simply want to raise a number of questions about the implications of this for the constitution of the 'British people'. Let us begin with the EU.

7.2.1   Citizenship of the European Union

We have already seen that being a 'citizen' means having a series of rights, entitlements and freedoms guaranteed by a state. No less is true of the status of citizen of the EU. The Maastricht Treaty is the document which sets out the rights EU citizens have. Drawing on work which sought to identify the hallmarks of citizenship (Gardner, 1994), Guild (1996) has compared the rights and duties of European citizenship against these hallmarks. A version of this is reproduced in Table 3.2.

Table 3.2 Citizenship of the European Union

	Hallmarks of citizenship	*Comparison with citizenship of the EU*
1	Freedom of movement; right to reside, to travel freely within the territory, to leave, to enter	EU citizens have the right to move and reside freely within the territory of the member states
2	Right to a passport	No right to a passport exists. A unified document was introduced requiring uniform design but issue and withdrawal conditions apparently remain a national prerogative
3	Entitlement to welfare benefits (including the right to housing)/obligation to contribution to social security systems	Treaty provides for the approximation of rules on social security so that migrant citizens of the Union are not penalized as regards social security rights by reason of their movement. Social security here means risk-related benefits. Social assistance benefits designed to keep people from poverty are not included.
		However, social assistance benefits must be made available on a non-discriminatory basis once the citizen of the Union has worked.
		Citizens of the Union are entitled to non-discrimination in respect of housing at least where they are exercising economic activities
4	The right to medical treatment/old age care	Where a citizen of the Union is engaged in an economic activity he or she must be entitled to equal treatment in this area; the general right of residence for students is subject to a requirement to be covered by sickness insurance
5	Right to education/vocational training	Citizens of the Union are entitled to move to pursue studies; where they are exercising economic activities their family members are entitled to education and vocational training as are they themselves if unemployed on the same basis as 'own nationals'
6	Freedom to exercise profession of choice/ right to work	This is a fundamental EU freedom limited only by circumstances where the citizen would be exercising state power

7	Right to vote in national and local elections	All citizens of EU member states have the right to vote in local elections and European Parliament elections. No right to vote in national (state) elections in countries where they reside but do not derive their citizenship from
8	Eligibility to stand as a candidate in national and local elections	Citizens of EU member states also have the right to stand for election in local and European Parliament elections
9	Right to petition and vote in referenda	The right to petition the European Ombudsman; access to bring a complaint to the European Parliament Committee of Petitions also exists
10	Access to justice: civil claims, administrative matters; entitlement to legal aid	Discrimination prohibited on the basis of nationality within the field of application of the treaty. Therefore the right of access to justice must be available on the same basis as for 'own nationals' as above
11	Liability to taxation	The EU tax – VAT – exists. As a tax on goods and services changing hands in the Union it applies to all persons in the Union
12	Allegiance to country of citizenship	Indeterminate in Union law

Note: there were 18 hallmarks which Guild compared – here I have only included those relevant to the concerns raised in this chapter.
Source: adapted from Guild, 1996, pp.47–9

The creation of the status of citizen of the EU with clearly defined rights and obligations raises a question about the extent to which it marks a move towards the separation or convergence of nationality and citizenship. In this case 'nationality' is to be understood as belonging to a specific nation in a cultural sense, and citizenship is to be understood as entitlements and duties within a specific state. As already noted, in legal terms it was only in the 1981 Nationality Act that the status of British citizen was established, but this Act did not define what it meant to be a British national. Somewhat paradoxically, given the ambivalent attitude of successive British governments towards the EU, what it means to be a 'British national' is defined solely in terms of the EU (Guild, 1996, p.32), and then only in a legal sense.

Despite this lack of legal definition and the existence of parallel citizenships for citizens of the member states of the EU, it is, however, doubtful that a separation between 'citizenship' and 'nationality' is occurring in terms of the rights and entitlements accruing to EU residents.

There are two reasons for reaching this conclusion. First, it remains the case that citizenship of the EU is fundamentally tied to the citizenship of a member state of the Union. So being a citizen of the UK, Germany or France, for example, is a precondition for being a citizen of the EU. This leads Martiniello (1994, p.35) to note that 'In its present shape, European citizenship is thus a sort of complementary supra-citizenship which confirms the existence of the cultural and political identities corresponding to the member states of the European Union.'

A second way to illustrate the continuing link between citizenship and nationality within the EU is in relation to the categorization of EU residents. Residents of the EU are divided into citizens, denizens and migrants, each with very different social, political and civil rights within the member states of the Union. Citizens living within the member state which grants them their citizenship/nationality have full rights. However, even these citizens have some restrictions on their full citizenship if they are resident within another state of the EU. As we saw in point 3 of Table 3.2, there is some limit on the extent to which citizens of one member state have full access to social security. This implies that the freedom of movement within the Union is restricted to those citizens with financial independence. Indeed, Martiniello (1994, p.41) has interpreted this as an attempt to limit the movement of the unemployed from states with a relatively lower level of social protection to those with relatively higher levels of such protection.

'Denizens' is the term used for legal residents of the EU who have 'third country' nationality but have some degree of civil and social rights. Generally speaking, their political rights are more limited. Moreover, as Read and Simpson (1991, p.30) have noted, when such people move across the borders of member states their rights often disappear, effectively transforming them into 'migrants'. This last category of EU residents – that is, migrants – is the group with few or no rights of citizenship, especially in relation to freedom of movement.

It is in the context of this hierarchical classification of the residents of the EU member states that the idea of 'Fortress Europe' and its associated system of immigration control arises. The concern to limit the numbers and rights of those defined either as 'Other' to Europeans or as second-class Europeans requires that the external borders of the Union are closed and heavily policed. It is an issue which continually tests the limits of the Union (and other smaller groupings within it) as the *Financial Times* article, partially reproduced below, makes clear.

Bavaria attacks Italy over Kurdish influx

By James Blitz in Rome

A German-Italian row over Kurdish refugees deepened yesterday when the southern German state of Bavaria accused Italy of irresponsibly expecting Germany to take care of hundreds of Kurds landing on the Italian coastline.

'More than half of all the people who come to Europe want to live in Germany because the law is more liberal and welfare payments are higher than in other countries,' said Günther Beckstein, Bavaria's interior minister.

...

The Italian government yesterday continued to come under pressure from its EU partners to strengthen its borders so that it can stem the intake of refugees. ...

(*Financial Times*, 8 January 1998, p.2)

Thus it seems that there is little evidence of a separation between nationality and citizenship in the EU. As a category of social rights and cultural belonging, then, the development of citizenship within the context of the EU seems to be no more inclusive than the construction of 'citizenship' at other moments in the

UK's history. It still acts as the means by which to construct boundaries of belonging and entitlement and thus is partially constitutive of a nationally and narrowly defined 'we'. The mirror image of this is to construct a series of 'Others' who occupy a range of subordinated citizenship statuses.

7.2.2 Devolution in the UK

If the formation of the status of citizenship of the EU expanded the geographical scope in which questions of citizenship could be discussed, events within the UK in 1997 pushed geographical parameters in the opposite direction. The event referred to is that of the votes in Wales and Scotland in favour of some form of devolution. The form this will take varies quite considerably in the two cases – with that in Scotland leading to a more pronounced form of devolution or regional self-government. The details of these are beyond the scope of this chapter's concerns, but what they do raise is the question of what it will mean in the future to talk about citizenship of the UK. Similarly, do the votes for devolution in Wales and Scotland indicate a strengthening or broadening of the sense of a national identity separate from that conjured up by the term 'British'? What forms of ethical connection or belonging do people in these two countries feel they have with people in England? As we have seen, all these are questions deeply connected to the idea of citizenship. We can also see that, in this sense, the language and imagery of citizenship is still central to the formation of a national popular. However, the vote, in 1997, in favour of Scottish and Welsh devolution, and the on-going peace process in Northern Ireland, alert us to the idea that who and what comprises the national popular is in constant negotiation. What the peace process and these votes indicated, especially that in Scotland where 80 per cent voted for a Scottish Assembly with the power to raise taxes, is that the *idea* of the UK as an 'imagined community' of belonging is, at the very least, subject to redefinition. Of course, at the time of writing we do not know the effects these processes will have on the constitution of a national identity – either in the UK as a whole, or in its constituent parts. What *is* clear is that the UK as a state has a population in which there are myriad, complex and competing identities at play. Each of these overlaps with numerous others making both far broader and far narrower boundaries of belonging. The extent to which the language and imagery of citizenship will emerge in the twenty-first century as the dominant sign through which 'the people' are connected – to each other, to the state and to welfare services – remains to be seen.

8 Conclusion

A number of more general points have been raised by our discussion of gendered and racial/national exclusions and subordinations which were a feature of British citizenship in the twentieth century. We have seen that, despite the formal equality of individuals who share a common citizenship, there are deep tensions between the social and individual aspects of citizenship, and that the limits to citizenship arise from the inequalities associated with particular social positions. The formal equality of citizenship does not prevent the marginalizations and exclusions which derive from membership of a subordinated group. Indeed, as we have seen, the actual operations of citizenship, both materially and symbolically, may be premised upon and reproduce these exclusions and subordinations.

It is this tension that Mouffe (1993) has suggested poses a major challenge to the liberal conception of citizenship and underlies how it might be possible to rethink the notion of citizenship in the context of social pluralism. One way of thinking about this would be in terms of how to construct another 'we'. As we have already seen, some argue for a series of 'I's who then constitute a 'we' by not making demands on 'the public' and engaging in forms of voluntary activity – examples are the arguments found in the All Party Parliamentary Report (HMSO, 1990) and in Green (1993), discussed in sections 4 and 5. Others want a 'we' formed out of a series of overlapping collectivities who continually reshape the 'we' in the context of constant political debate – for example, Purdy (1994) and Fraser (1997), discussed in sections 5 and 6.1 respectively. Thus we have also seen that citizenship is a deeply political process – that is, its character, limits and entitlements are formed within an endless process of contestation and negotiation. On the cusp of the twenty-first century how the 'we' is constituted and what entitlements and duties accrue to those who claim citizenship in the UK is at the centre of public debate. Moreover, this debate occurs in the context of the UK's membership of the EU and its changing relationship with the Commonwealth.

Further reading

There is a huge literature on citizenship available, but the work by T.H. Marshall listed in the References below offers a good starting-point for those interested in pursuing further the issues raised here. The titles by Andrews (1991), Barbalet (1988), Bauböck (1994), Cesarani and Fulbrook (1996), Paul (1997), Taylor (1996) and Yuval-Davis (1997) are also helpful for exploring questions of inclusion and exclusion associated with citizenship status. Two further texts are also useful additions to this list. These are: Roche (1992), which explores the philosophical roots in traditional notions of citizenship and investigates possible reformulations; and *Feminist Review* (1997), which provides insights into current feminist thinking about the potential and limitations of citizenship for transcending relations of inequality in various nation-states.

References

Andrews, G. (ed.) (1991) *Citizenship*, London, Lawrence and Wishart.

Barbalet, J.M. (1988) *Citizenship, Rights, Struggle and Class Inequality*, Milton Keynes, Open University Press.

Bauböck, R. (ed.) (1994) *From Aliens to Citizens: Redefining the Status of Immigrants in Europe*, Aldershot, Avebury.

Cesarani, D. (1996) 'The changing character of citizenship and nationality in Britain', in Cesarani and Fulbrook (eds) (1996).

Cesarani, D. and Fulbrook, M. (eds) (1996) *Citizenship, Nationality and Migration in Europe*, London, Routledge.

Cochrane, A. (1998) 'What sort of safety-net? Social security, income maintenance and the benefits system', in Hughes and Lewis (eds) (1998).

Colley, L. (1992) *Britons: Forging the Nation 1707–1837*, Newhaven, CT and London, Yale University Press.

Commission for Racial Equality (1985) *Immigration Control Procedures*, London, Commission for Racial Equality.

Dummett, A. (1994) 'The acquisition of British citizenship, from imperial traditions to national definitions', in Baubóck (ed.) (1994).

Dwyer, C. (1993) 'Constructions of Muslim identity and the contesting of power: the debate over Muslim schools in the UK', in Jackson, P. and Penrose, J. (eds) *Constructions of Race, Place and Nation*, London, UCL Press.

Feminist Review (1997) 'Citizenship: pushing the boundaries', *Feminist Review*, 57.

Forgacs, D. (1993) 'National-popular: genealogy of a concept', in During, S. (ed.) *Cultural Studies Reader*, London, Routledge.

Fraser, N. (1997) 'After the family wage: a postindustrial thought experiment', in Fraser, N. (ed.) *Justice Interruptus: Critical Reflections on the 'Postsocialist' Condition*, New York, Routledge.

Gardner, J.P. (ed.) (1994) *Hallmarks of Citizenship: A Green Paper*, London, British Institute of International and Comparative Law.

Gorz, A. (1992) 'On the difference between society and community and why basic income cannot by itself confer membership of either' in van Parijs (ed.) (1992).

Gramsci, A. (1971) *Selections from the Prison Notebooks*, London, Lawrence and Wishart.

Green, D.G. (1993) *Reinventing Civil Society: The Rediscovery of Welfare Without Politics*, London, Institute of Economic Affairs.

Guild, E. (1996) 'The legal framework of citizenship of the European Union', in Cesarani and Fulbrook (eds) (1996).

Held, D. (1991) 'Between state and civil society: citizenship', in Andrews (ed.) (1991).

Hickman, M.J. (1998) 'Reconstructing and deconstructing "race": British political discourses about the Irish in Britain', in *Ethnic and Racial Studies*, vol.21, no.2.

HMSO (1990) *Encouraging Citizenship*, Report of the Commission on Citizenship, London, HMSO.

Hughes, G. (1998) '"Picking over the remains": the welfare state settlements of the post-Second World War UK', in Hughes and Lewis (eds) (1998).

Hughes, G. and Lewis, G. (eds) (1998) *Unsettling Welfare: The Reconstruction of Social Policy*, London, Routledge in association with The Open University.

Jordan, B. (1992) 'Basic income and community' in van Parijs (ed.) (1992).

Langan, M. (1998) 'The contested concept of need', in Langan, M. (ed.) *Welfare: Needs, Rights and Risks*, London, Routledge in association with The Open University.

Leca, J. (1991) 'Individualisme et citoyennete', in Birnbaum, P. and Leca, J. (eds) *Sur l'Individualisme*, Paris, Presses de la Fondation Nationale des Sciences Politiques.

Lewis, G. (1998a) '"Coming apart at the seams": the crises of the welfare state', in Hughes and Lewis (eds) (1998).

Lewis, G. (1998b) 'Review' in Lewis (ed.) (1998c).

Lewis, G. (ed.) (1998c) *Forming Nation: Framing Welfare*, London, Routledge in association with The Open University.

Marshall, T.H. (1981a) 'Welfare in the context of social policy', in Marshall (ed.) (1981c).

Marshall, T.H. (1981b) 'The right to welfare', in Marshall (ed.) (1981c).

Marshall, T.H. (1981c) *The Right to Welfare and Other Essays*, London, Heinemann.

Marshall, T.H. (1996) 'Citizenship and social class' (first published in 1950), in Marshall, T.H. and Bottomore, T. (eds) *Citizenship and Social Class*, London, Pluto.

Martiniello, M. (1994) 'Citizenship of the European Union: a critical view', in Bauböck (ed.) (1994).

McCoy, L. (1998) 'Education for labour: social problems of nationhood', in Lewis (ed.) (1998c).

Miller, D. (1995) 'Reflections on British national identity', *New Community*, vol.21, no.2, pp.153–66.

Mouffe, C. (1993) 'Liberal socialism and pluralism: which citizenship?', in Squires, J. (ed.) *Principled Positions, Postmodernism and the Rediscovery of Value*, London, Lawrence and Wishart.

Pascall, G. (1993) 'Citizenship – a feminist analysis', in Drover, G. and Kerans, P. (eds) *New Approaches to Welfare Theory*, Aldershot, Edward Elgar.

Paul, K. (1997) *Whitewashing Britain: Race and Citizenship in the Postwar Era*, Ithaca, NY, Cornell University Press.

Purdy, D. (1994) 'Citizenship, basic income and the state', *New Left Review*, no.208, pp.30–48.

Read, M. and Simpson, A. (1991) *Against a Rising Tide: Racism, Europe and 1992*, London, Spokesman.

Roche, M. (1992) *Rethinking Citizenship*, Cambridge, Polity.

Silverman, M. (1996) 'The revenge of civil society: state, nation and society in France', in Cesarani and Fulbrook (eds) (1996).

Taylor. D. (1996) 'Citizenship and social power', in Taylor, D. (ed.) *Critical Social Policy – A Reader, Social Policy and Social Relations*, London, Sage.

van Parijs, P. (ed.) (1992) *Arguments for Basic Income*, Verso, London.

Yuval-Davis, N. (1997) *Gender and Nation*, London, Sage.

CHAPTER 4

Reinventing 'the Public'?

by Gordon Hughes, John Clarke, Gail Lewis and Gerry Mooney

Contents

1   Introduction

This book has concentrated on the imaginary figures of welfare that have emerged following the break-up of the social settlement associated with the social democratic welfare state in the post-war UK (see **Hughes and Lewis, 1998**). The Introduction argued that the 1980s and 1990s had witnessed an onslaught on the social democratic notion of 'the public', partly arising from the contradictions, uncertainties and ambiguities of the Beveridgean social settlement. The result was a collapse of the dominant representation of the people, 'the public' and the state, a representation that we have called 'the social democratic national popular'. This collapse provided the context in which different symbolic representations of the people and 'the public' were articulated as competing conceptions of how social welfare could be remade. In Chapters 1, 2 and 3 we explored three ways of reimagining the possible relationships between individuals, the state and social welfare in the late twentieth century. All three figures – the consumer, the community and the citizen – are arguably haunted by the unresolved social settlement in the post-welfare state era (what we might call 'the ghosts of settlements past'). Furthermore, all three contain complex and volatile meanings and, in a profound sense, are unfinished.

This book has explored the competing ideological positions and multi-faceted, complex debates on the possible futures of social welfare. The main aims of this review chapter are to offer you:

- an overview of the main themes, concepts and debates of the book;
- a review of the main debates in each of the three chapters on the new imaginary figures of welfare – the consumer, community and citizen;
- an understanding of the ways in which the representations around consumer, community and citizen are linked to broader debates on the future relationships between social welfare, the state and 'the public';
- a critical grasp of welfare as an object of continuing political and ideological controversy.

1.1   The assault on 'the public'

The Introduction to this book contained an overview of what we have termed the assault on 'the public' during the 1980s and 1990s.

ACTIVITY 4.1

Look back over the Introduction quickly and think about the following questions:

1   What were the main features of the assault on 'the public'?

2   What were the main consequences of this assault for the nature of social welfare in the UK in the 1980s and 1990s?

3   In what ways did the old social settlement come apart?

COMMENT

The Introduction pointed to an ideological attack on the post-war welfare state that focused on its expense and its role in creating welfare dependency. We suggested that 'the public' may be defined as something that identified the intersection of the people/welfare/state. This definition allows for the fact that the meaning of the terms 'people', 'welfare' and 'state' are changing, as are the ways in which the three terms are linked together. There was a shift from what is often termed social democratic welfarism – that is, state-based forms of social provision involving some redistributive justice, based partly on contributions and partly on needs – to more marketized, entrepreneurial, consumerist forms of organization and representation (see **Hughes and Lewis, 1998**).

■ ■ ■

The Introduction also pointed to evidence of multiple disaffections with the old Beveridgean welfare state. These criticisms and challenges were associated with the voices from the margins of the old social settlement, such as anti-racist groups, the disability movement and feminists. They coincided with the New Right's critique of the (welfare) state and celebration of the market (**Lewis, 1998b**). Two particular aspects of these challenges were important:

1   the implosion – or collapsing inwards – of the social democratic settlement under the weight of its own contradictions;

2   the collapse of the distinction between 'the natural' and 'the social' that had allowed the social democratic welfare state to deal with social justice and inequality as matters of class only.

We noted that the combined effort to redefine 'natural' distinctions into social divisions helped to undermine the social settlement of the Beveridgean welfare state.

Given these challenges to the Beveridgean welfare state, we may ask ourselves who were the winners. Arguably, the welfare system in the UK which resulted from the changes of the last two decades of the twentieth century was meaner, narrower, more miserable and more privatized than that which developed between the 1940s and the 1970s. But this is not the same as saying that the New Right won. Instead, we suggested that two things happened simultaneously:

1   The debates covered in this book operate on political and social landscapes that have been profoundly shaped by the New Right (though there are important degrees of social and geographical unevenness across the UK). Indicative of the victory of the New Right was the shift to a discourse of managers, markets and privatization in place of one that featured public servants, state planning and public ownership. This shift has taken place alongside the growth, and greater acceptance, of inequalities in an 'enterprise culture'.

2   The New Right or Thatcherite conception of the people as individuals and consumers rather than members of a collective public did not triumph but remained profoundly contested. It would appear that much of the success of the Labour Party in the 1997 General Election was related to a broad dissatisfaction with the New Right's denial of the 'social', most famously expressed in Margaret Thatcher's claim that there is no such thing as society, only individuals and their families.

1.2   Representing 'the public'

It will be evident that the assault on 'the public' was as much about the struggle of ideas and representations as it was about changing organizations and institutional practices. This is self-consciously a book about ideas, visions and representations – about 'how it is all thought and talked about' – rather than a book about the institutional and organizational arrangements of social welfare. (On the restructuring of the welfare state see **Hughes and Lewis, 1998**.) The Introduction gave some attention to what is meant by ideas of representations and imaginary relations of welfare. **Lewis (1998a)** suggested that it is helpful to think of 'the imaginary' as the means by which human beings attempt to give some order and logic to – or make sense of – the diverse range of activities they engage in by creating names, categorizations and normative standards. Such attempts to create order include nineteenth-century notions of 'the nation' and distinctions between the deserving and undeserving poor, as well as contemporary appeals to the people as either rational, self-seeking calculators in the market place or altruistic members of 'a community'.

This book has demonstrated that there is a rich representational dimension to contemporary debates around social welfare, and that the contested understandings of where welfare may be heading are themselves deeply enmeshed in wider notions of what it means to be 'British', 'different' or 'responsible'. They also connect with conflicting views about what is the appropriate and proper relationship of the people to the state, market or institutions of civil society. As Chapter 3, section 1.1 noted, the national popular represents 'a means of constructing a "we"'. The preceding chapters traced attempts to reinvent a social order, and to redefine who belongs to it as well as who is excluded. The Introduction argued that figures and visions associated with the consumer, the community and the citizen represent contested attempts to reconstruct a national popular. In one sense all three visions relate to questions of *who* gets connected and *how* they get connected. At the same time, all three figures relate to questions of *who* gets disconnected and *how* they get disconnected. Such questions lie at the heart of the contemporary debate over social inclusions and exclusions. To put it differently, these figures conjure up imageries of people who are 'us' distinguished from people who are not 'us', but are the 'Other'.

2   Articulating new figures of welfare

Chapters 1, 2 and 3 traced three attempts to refigure or reconstruct the subjects of welfare. In this section we review the main themes of these chapters and the major points of tension associated with them. Consumer, community and citizen are not one-dimensional or wholly unified figures or visions; they are subject to conflicting interpretations. So, while these chapters examined the focal points of each figure, they also alerted you to the debates around these focal points. All three figures represent discursive points around which are articulated imaginary relationships between the people, the state and social welfare. In turn they help us explore the socially constructed character of welfare belongings, entitlements and duties, and exclusions. For example, Chapter 2 outlined two very different discourses on community, one associated with moral communitarianism and the other with radical left pluralism. For the former, the idea of community involves a powerful appeal to an exclusive, bounded entity within which people are naturally and hierarchically ordered. For the latter, communities are viewed as processes in the making, without any abiding 'essences', often resulting from struggles for the acceptance of difference and the fight against oppression. Noting these different positions on the figure of community should not, however, prevent us from recognizing some focal points shared by commentators of both the Right and Left. In particular, the language of reciprocity, solidarity, mutuality and the idea of balancing rights and obligations cuts across the discourses of both moral communitarians and radical left pluralists. Another focal point shared by both sides was the opposition to what Hughes and Mooney (Chapter 2, section 4) described as 'statist forms of social policy and welfare organization'. We saw that community was positioned as somewhere between the state and the individual, a position that underpins its seductive capacity to gain support from across the political and ideological spectrum.

Think back to the debates around the consumer and the citizen in Chapters 1 and 3 and try to note examples of how these two figures, like community, are subject to contested constructions. Are there any shared focal points for each of these two figures?

2.1 Welfare subjects as consumers

Chapter 1 focused on the dominant discourse which emerged out of the crisis of the Beveridgean settlements, namely consumerism, based on the image of the individual in the market place. In the discourse of neo-liberalism, consumerism is linked to the promotion of the enterprise culture and the supremacy of the market as the institution for delivering both wealth and welfare. But it was also evident that other voices see consumerism as a potential means of empowerment of the marginalized and oppressed. Nevertheless, these other voices were relatively marginal compared with the dominant neo-liberal meanings of consumerism that stress the capacity of individual consumers to exercise power.

ACTIVITY 4.2

Consider the following questions about the relationship of consumerism to power relations:

1   What form of power does market-based consumerism create?
2   What are the strengths and limitations of this form of power in relation to social welfare?

COMMENT

Market-based consumerism is associated with economic power: the economic capacity (buying power) of individuals, households or organizations determines the influence and range of choices they can exercise. In relation to social welfare, there are two problems about this form of consumerism. The first concerns whether it is *possible* to create effective markets for welfare benefits and services, such that people can exercise consumer choice. The second concerns whether it is *desirable* to have markets and consumerism in social welfare, because of their unwanted economic, social and political consequences.

■ ■ ■

2.2   Welfare subjects as members of communities

Chapter 2 examined discourses around community as contested ways of imagining the relationship of the people to 'the public', the state and social welfare. The chapter stressed the slippery and elusive nature of the notion of community in both common-sense usage and understanding and in debates in the social sciences. The discussion also drew attention to the immensely powerful and seductive character of the notion of community. The chapter went on to outline two starkly contrasting discourses on community: moral communitarianism, the dominant discourse on community in the UK in the late twentieth century, and radical left pluralism, the more peripheral discourse during this period. It was emphasized that the dominant moral communitarian discourse carried distinctly conservative, 'naturalizing' notions of how 'we' should live our lives, not least in terms of the delivery, organization and responsibility for social welfare.

Think about the place occupied by the family in the moral communitarian discourse on social welfare. What assumptions does this discourse make about the family? How does it view the role of the family?

In their discourse on welfare, Etzioni (1994; 1995), Dennis (1993a, b; 1997), Phillips (1996) and Green (1996) give a central and privileged place to the family (in the singular). The family is viewed as the natural and essential site in which to establish and pass on the 'normal' ways of being in the social world. In turn, people are differently and hierarchically positioned as welfare subjects according to their 'natures' (woman as mother and carer, man as wage-earning breadwinner and authority figure, child as dependent). More generally, this conservative variant of communitarianism articulated a 'moral obligations over legal rights' discourse on family matters. Voluntarism and self-help are celebrated – not least through the institution of the family – as the most natural means of delivering welfare, with the role of the state limited largely to controlling and regulating the 'pathological' and deviant households of the 'underclass'.

The radical left pluralists offer a different vision of the future of social welfare. According to this discourse nothing is fixed by nature or tradition; the notion of communit*ies* is one of constant process and struggle.

Why is there an emphasis in radical left pluralism on the use of the plural term 'communities' rather than the singular 'community'?

Radical left pluralists see the process of forging imagined communities as both a source of activism and a source of making (welfare) demands on the state or the public agencies, as in examples such as the campaigns and self-organizations of gay and lesbian people and lone parents, cited by Weeks (1996) and Pahl (1995), and disabled people (**Hughes, 1998a**).

2.3 Welfare subjects as citizens

Chapter 3 began by examining the classic social democratic position articulated by T.H. Marshall (1996) on the citizen as the subject of social welfare in modern society. This construction of the citizen, embodied in the white, British, male, able-bodied worker/father/husband, was the central figure in the imagery of the social democratic welfare state. The chapter then examined the intense ideological struggles in the late twentieth century over the meaning of the term citizen, arguing that these struggles were both internal to and outside of the 'British nation'.

What contradictions and ambiguities were identified in Chapter 3 around this image of the citizen?

The chapter plotted how the figure of the citizen could not hold the contradictions within it. It embodied the myth of universalism and unity, linked to the notion of the supposedly homogeneous British 'race', and hid both the realities of profoundly unequal power relations and the extent and forms of social diversity. It thus generated its own boundaries of belonging and outsiderness, in particular, constructing positions of second-class citizenship for subordinated welfare subjects. Chapter 3 then explored the emergent plural and non-national imaginings of citizenships that emerged from the shattering of the social democratic figure of the citizen. These took the form of new articulations, such as those arising from feminist critiques and expressed by writers such as Pascall (1993) and Fraser (1997) (Chapter 3, section 6). Pascall in particular focused on the disjuncture between formal political equality and substantive inequality between the sexes in all three elements of the 'Marshallian' discourse. The discussion of the work of Fraser moved beyond that of the critique of existing relations to explicit imaginings of a Utopian future based on the 'Universal Caregiver' welfare state in which the gendered opposition between breadwinning and caregiving would be dismantled. This project for a new national popular would thus entail the deconstruction of dominant gender norms.

There were multiple challenges to the social democratic notion of the citizen. Alongside the feminist challenges there were important contestations around the links between 'nation' and 'race'. We saw that the unravelling of the notion of the British (imperial) citizen raised new possibilities for reimagining citizenship beyond the borders of the nation, and for challenging the racialized discourse of 'British subjects' and 'aliens' inscribed in legislation throughout the twentieth century.

Two key questions remained from this debate on citizenship. First, how might the struggles and voices of what was termed the 'Other' necessitate a new discourse of citizen rights? Second, will the supra-national state associated with the European Union open up spaces for the renegotiation of the meanings of citizenship? Chapter 3 provides powerful evidence of the multiple struggles that take place *within* each vision as well as between the three figures.

2.4 Reinventing the people: what sort of nation?

Consumer, community and citizen all offer potential new 'subject positions' (**Lewis, 1998b**) through which people may come to see themselves and think of themselves in new ways. Arguably all three have both attractions and limitations as visions of the future of social welfare and for what it might mean to be a member of 'the public'.

Think back over the discussions in Chapters 1, 2 and 3 and jot down the particular appeals of the discourses on the consumer, the community and the citizen.

COMMENT

We discuss the appeals, as well as some of the problems, of the three discourses below. Here, we want to underline the point that discourses work by trying to construct subject positions that people can identify with, or that they can see themselves in. All three of the discourses try to construct positions for 'us', and try to make them appear attractive positions for 'us' to occupy.

■ ■ ■

Let us now look at the three discourses in turn. We have tried to sketch what each of them offers as a construction of 'the people' and how each of those constructions might appeal.

2.4.1   A nation of consumers?

In the neo-liberal discourse on consumerism there is the powerful, seemingly obvious, appeal of the consumerist 'democracy' of the market. Being a consumer is how we may commonsensically see ourselves in some aspects of our lives, such as in the routine activities of shopping or being a tourist. Being positioned as a consumer in the context of social welfare appears to offer us choice and empowerment in contrast to being dependent on bureaucratic and professional experts who 'know best'. The discourse of consumerism may also open up new representational spaces, given the radical turn on consumerism and new local governance discussed in Chapter 1, section 3.2.

However, the dominant neo-liberal discourse on the consumer involves the valorization of the private realm over 'the public', with welfare to be funded by individuals making provision for themselves in appropriate market places. Furthermore, if the consumer cannot do this (by pursuing his or her own goals as a calculating and rational decision-maker in the market), it becomes the individual's fault. So the dominant discourse on consumerism carries a narrower view of 'the public' than the old social democratic vision. The figure of the consumer thus represents symbolically the dismantling of collective notions of 'the public' and their replacement by images of individualized users of services. The discourse of consumerism involves the simultaneous disempowerment of the collective vision of 'the public' and a process of qualified and selective empowerment of people as individual consumers, since not all people can 'consume' successfully.

2.4.2   A nation of communities?

Chapter 2 argued that the 'rediscovery of community' in the 1980s and 1990s emerged in reaction to the impoverishment of the public realm effected by New Right ideology and policy. It also argued that the notion of community in the conservative discourse of moral communitarianism is often nostalgic and thus problematic, calling on mythic and idealized sets of images of the people as homogeneous, as in the portrayal of traditional British working class communities as solid, supportive and orderly. There is an at times implicit, at other times explicit, rallying call to a moral community as the site of the self-provision of welfare, with the cult of familialism, involving the celebration of an idealized, 'traditional family' at its heart.

The more radical visions of community, associated with radical left pluralism, view communities as 'necessary fictions' to be struggled for, but remaining forever unfinished. As Weeks (1996, p.83) notes, with regard to the idea of the sexual community of gays and lesbians, 'it is a necessary fiction because it offers the possibility of social agency in a context where equal access to social goods is denied.'

Throughout the discussion of the moral communitarian and radical left pluralist discourses, tensions were evident between notions of community as territory, geographical locality or shared cultural identity versus communities of interests and affiliations and communities as processes of collective struggles. Both discourses acknowledge the appeal of community in that it seems to address the sense of loss created by the Thatcherite claim that there is no such thing as society. There is, therefore, some shared ideological ground on the importance of 'the social' and 'the communal' across the major ideological divide between moral communitarianism and radical left pluralism. The appeal of, and to, community may thus revitalize notions of a civil society that is not reducible to the state or market place. But it also accords with what we have termed the assault on 'the public'. This is manifested most strikingly in government strategies that put the responsibility for delivering social welfare and alleviating social harms on to 'the community' rather than the state. Specific examples of this include the development of informal networks for the provision of social care and self-help crime prevention schemes such as Neighbourhood Watch.

2.4.3 A nation of citizens?

Citizenship broadly embodies a set of rights which are held by the citizen in relation to the state. The social democratic vision offered to many people a clear sense of belonging to a wider public body – the nation/state. This belonging was based on rights and obligations. However, Chapter 3 raised the crucial question of whether the figure of the citizen could be reforged without producing exclusions around such categories as the nation, class, 'race', gender and able-bodiedness. Historically the concept of citizenship has been characterized by what Chapter 3, section 3 termed 'its own boundaries of belonging and outsiderness'. In the Marshallian notion of the citizen it was obvious that the basis for social citizenship was gendered (**Morris, 1998**). This social democratic citizen subject was also associated with a clearly bounded and exclusionary notion of the nation, determining who, on the basis of racialized inclusions and exclusions, was an 'insider' or an 'alien'.

Chapter 3 explored the ways in which the challenges to the limitations of the social democratic construction of citizenship had opened up new possibilities. In relation to the structuring implications of gender, 'race' and nation, new developments could be seen that created *expanded* varieties of citizenship, with new inclusions. In this respect, citizenship might go beyond 'a nation of citizens' to see citizenship rights, obligations and identities located in institutions beyond the nation state (in European structures, for example). By contrast with the other two discourses, however, citizenship remains firmly a *public* conception of the people. It is a figure that is self-consciously located in people's relationships with public and political institutions.

3 Contextualizing the seductions of the consumer, community and citizen

In section 2 we reviewed the key themes of each of the three imaginary figures. We also reviewed how these figures were subject to varying, and politically volatile, ways of appropriating their meaning. These representational figures do not have a simple ideological or political pedigree, nor are they necessarily attached to any one *political project* of reconstructing the national popular. However, in this section we will be exploring the extent to which all three figures are framed within a common context in which new ways of thinking about the relationships between individuals and groups, the state, the market and welfare are being constructed. What is their place in reinventing 'the public'?

The main features of the political terrain in the UK and other Western capitalist societies at the end of the twentieth century were inherited from the New Right transformations of the economy, society and polity in the 1980s and 1990s. The long-term consequences of the market-like restructuring of social welfare and the public sphere are likely to mean that social welfare will be shaped by pressures to be more targeted, rationed and selective. The chapters in this book point to a process in which moral dimensions have become a significant part of the future of social welfare: an 'upping' of the moral nature of what 'the social' is, for example, in contested conceptions of responsibility, duty and desert. The three figures of consumer, community and citizen have all been employed in a reassertion of the virtues of self-reliance and a rejection of state paternalism as a means of realizing social welfare (see Smith, 1997). This new moral regime about who gets, should get, and how they get welfare has been viewed by some commentators as involving a specific 'register of [moral] blame' (Rustin, 1997, p.10).

In this process, individuals – in families, in communities, and as 'active citizens' – have been required to take more responsibility for their welfare and well-being. This development is in line with the move towards what has been termed 'governance at a distance', which tries to reduce the state's responsibilities for social welfare (Rhodes, 1997). In particular, stressing individual responsibility draws attention away from the state's active role in defining and repositioning the boundary between the public and the private (Clarke and Newman, 1997, Chapter 1). It is important, therefore, not to lose sight of the changing nature of state power in any emergent settlements around welfare. In the emergent political settlement of the late twentieth century, the state is no longer viewed as the primary provider of welfare. Rather its role appears to be to engage with a range of diverse organizations, families and individuals in the production and distribution of social welfare. The reshaping of the public/private divide is thus a complex process in which we see withdrawal of the state in some ways and extension of its influence in others (see **Clarke *et al.*, 1998**).

One way of exploring the differences between the discourses of consumer, community and citizen is to imagine how they each might respond to particular social policy initiatives or proposals. For example, in 1998 there were discussions about introducing a curfew on children, with the intention that children should not be out in the street later than early evening. The policy was presented as a way of (a) protecting children; (b) protecting 'the public'; and (c) reinforcing the family and parental authority. How do you think each of the three discourses might address this policy? Which of them might favour it and why?

COMMENT

A curfew on children seems most likely to appeal to, and be supported by arguments from, the moral communitarian strand in the *community* discourse. The policy could be seen as a means of remoralizing the community, restoring family responsibilities and strengthening traditional forms of authority. The radical left pluralist version of community might, however, point to the intrusive, statist character of such a policy.

In relation to *citizenship*, the policy raises some difficult issues. It appears to emphasize some sorts of citizenship rights (citizens being protected from potential nuisance or crime) and enforces some obligations (the responsibilities of parents). However, it raises problems about the limits and exclusions it constructs in relation to citizenship. In defining children as not having the right to be in public places, does it create a basis for treating one set of people in terms that could not be applied to others? Does it, indeed, exclude children from citizenship rights?

It is not clear that a *consumerist* discourse would have much to say about a curfew on children. There may be questions of how it should be funded: by all residents; a levy on parents; a contribution from those who want to be protected from children? There may also be questions about how it should be implemented: by the police; or contracted out to a private agency? There is also the issue of who the potential consumers of such a policy would be: all residents of an area (or at least all adult residents); all parents, or just the parents of children picked up under the policy? Can the children themselves be consumers of the service?

■ ■ ■

A thread running through this book is the attempt to create (and criticize) what in some ways is a new moral discourse, but one that involves going 'back to the future'. There are elements of nineteenth-century notions in which excluded, marginalized and undeserving 'others' are distinguished from included, deserving, responsible and active members of the welfare community (**Morris, 1998**). We have seen that such ideas as 'choice', 'need', 'right' and 'obligation' can be used as the focus for the campaigning efforts of particular groups, as a means of articulating and making demands on the welfare system. They are also ways of defining 'we' and 'others' as recognizable social groupings. Such terms and the social distinctions they construct are resisted and fought against through other representations. It is clear, then, that the figures of the consumer, the community and the citizen carry notions of *normalization*: that is, they are prescriptive about, as well as descriptive of, how we live and belong to social orders and how needs, entitlements and obligations are distributed. Such norms matter, because as 'the injunctions about what ought to be, what is best, what is natural, [they] serve to mark the boundaries of inclusion and exclusion' (**Lewis, 1998a, p.31**).

4   A new social settlement?

Is there a new social settlement? In other words, are there any new norms about the contemporary forms of the ideological trinity – Family, Work and Nation – of the old Beveridgean social settlement (Williams, 1989; **Hughes, 1998b**)? This ideological trinity organized the formation of national identity ('race'), the familial divisions of labour (gender) and work–welfare linkages (class) into an imaginary field of naturalized identities which constructed the British people as citizens. The interaction of this set of ideological assumptions was crucial to the construction of the Beveridgean, social democratic welfare state in the post-war UK. Family and work interacted in assumptions about the organization of waged and unwaged work. There was also the precondition of some consensus with regard to the expanded role of the state in maintaining full male employment. Welfare needs were thus to be met through the earned income of the male head, while the family was viewed as a natural site of biological differences between men and women. There was also an assumption about the ethnicity of these citizens, that they were 'British-born white'. This resulted in the inscription of a singular set of patterns of life, values and needs at the heart of the welfare services *as if* they were universal.

Almost all political positions have agreed that there can be no going back to the Beveridgean welfare state, and that social welfare needed reform to match the demands of a changed and changing society. However, we suggested in Chapters 1, 2 and 3 that significant tensions continue around the discourses of welfare subjects as consumers, as providers within communities or as citizens. Some of these tensions have arisen from unresolved conflicts about the direction and character of social change. Are lone-parent families 'deviant', or a different form of household? In what ways is the UK a 'multi-ethnic' society? Has poverty deepened, or has an 'underclass' developed? What citizenship rights are denied to or claimed by gay and lesbian people? Questions such as these exemplify the unsettled and continuing disputes about what sort of society this *is* and *should be*.

Furthermore, there appeared in the last decades of the twentieth century to be both renewed celebration of, and contestation over, the family, with a stress on arguments for moral unity versus diversity to the fore. **Morris (1998)** pointed to the instability and breakdown of the 'old' family, work and nation nexus in the 1990s due to the decline of paid employment for men, the challenges to the nuclear family, and the attacks on the use of welfare to fill the breach. At the same time, Morris noted the lack of a viable alternative to the old settlement in which the role of work was vital to men's personal and social worth, while the traditional obligations of women revolved around home and family. It is also questionable whether there could be a new hegemonic norm about the nature of the nation given the diversity of the population of the UK. However, work as paid employment for all pre-retirement age adults appeared to have a central place in the emergent project of the New Labour government in the late 1990s. In fact, it was arguably its articulating principle. It seemed that all pre-retirement age citizens (including young people, mothers and disabled people), were to be persuaded, or coerced if necessary, into the realm of paid work, irrespective of gender. At the same time, it is important to note that work in this context of the late twentieth century did not mean the same thing as work in the old settlement: the conditions, careers and social distribution of paid work all underwent significant transformations in the last decades of the century (Flynn, 1994).

This attempt to reform, or 'modernize', the welfare state was dominated by the image of welfare to work, an image derived from US welfare policy (**Cochrane, 1998**). It contrasted the 'independence' that came from being in work with the problem of 'being dependent on benefits'. This image underpinned arguments about the need to reform welfare in the late 1990s. It exposed further tensions: the balance between the obligation to work and the obligation to care for their children for lone mothers; the apparently residualized status of those who could not find or take paid employment; and the financial and social costs of an increased reliance on means testing for welfare benefits and services. In their different ways these tensions marked the continuing uncertainty about the social settlement in relation to welfare.

5   Conclusion

The word 'conclusion' may be a misnomer in a book about looking forward, about possible futures. There remains much conflict about what may form a new social settlement. Our main concern has been to look at processes of reinventing 'the public'. It is clear that 'the public' is not a natural thing, but something constructed, deconstructed and reconstructed over time. The discourses around the consumer, the community and the citizen have articulated new representational spaces in which to position and see ourselves. All lay claim to being able to speak for the 'public interest'. While it is not clear what has replaced the old social democratic representations, it is clear that these old certainties (themselves not unproblematic nor uncontested) have been unlocked and loosened. At the same time, there have been attempts to reconstruct some forms of these old certainties, for example in the appeal to a 'return to community'. But such attempts have been partial and uncertain, while major tensions remain around the appeals to the people as consumers in markets, members of communities, or citizens as legal members of a political society.

When reading this book you may be aware of new debates and disputes around social welfare, but we are confident that it will be difficult to imagine any future in which the politics of representation and articulation around social welfare will not centre on the three figures of the consumer, the community and the citizen. As we have seen, discourses on social welfare are deeply enmeshed in the process of representing what the nation is and will be. The conflicting discourses of welfare that have emerged since the break-up of the old Beveridgean welfare state are also central to the operation of power and the processes of social exclusion and inclusion which emerge from it. 'The public' is clearly being remade, but its future shape will be decided only by the political struggles over contested representations.

References

Clarke, J., Hughes, G. and Lewis, G. (1998) 'Review', in Hughes and Lewis (eds) (1998).

Clarke, J. and Newman, J. (1997) *The Managerial State*, London, Sage.

Cochrane, A. (1998) 'What sort of safety-net? Social security, income maintenance and the benefits system', in Hughes and Lewis (eds) (1998).

Dennis, N. (1993a) *Rising Crime and the Dismembered Family*, London, Institute of Economic Affairs.

Dennis, N. (1993b) in Dennis, N. and Erdos, G. (eds) *Families Without Fatherhood*, London, Institute of Economic Affairs.

Dennis, N. (1997) *The Invention of Permanent Poverty*, London, Institute of Economic Affairs.

Etzioni, A. (1994) *The Spirit of Community: The Reinvention of American Society*, New York, Touchstone.

Etzioni, A. (1995) *The Spirit of Community: Rights, Responsibilities and the Communitarian Agenda*, London, Fontana.

Flynn, N. (1994) 'Control, commitment and contracts', in Clarke, J., Cochrane, A. and McLaughlin, E. (eds) *Managing Social Policy*, London, Sage.

Fraser, N. (1997) 'After the family wage: a postindustrial thought experiment', in Fraser, N. (ed.) *Justice Interruptus: Critical Reflections on the Postsocialist Condition*, New York, Routledge.

Green, D. (1996) *Community Without Politics: A Market Approach to Welfare Reform*, London, Institute of Economic Affairs.

Hughes, G. (1998a) 'A suitable case for treatment?: Constructions of disability', in Saraga, E. (ed.) *Embodying the Social: Constructions of Difference*, London, Routledge in association with The Open University.

Hughes, G. (1998b) '"Picking over the remains": the welfare state settlements of the post-Second World War UK', in Hughes and Lewis (eds) (1998).

Hughes, G. and Lewis, G. (eds) (1998) *Unsettling Welfare: The Reconstruction of Social Policy*, London, Routledge in association with The Open University.

Lewis, G. (1998a) 'Review', in Lewis, G. (ed.) *Forming Nation*, *Framing Welfare*, London, Routledge in association with The Open University.

Lewis, G. (1998b) '"Coming apart at the seams": the crisis of the welfare state', in Hughes and Lewis (eds) (1998).

Marshall, T.H. (1996) 'Citizenship and social class' (first published 1950), in Marshall, T.H. and Bottomore, T. (eds) *Citizenship and Social Class*, London, Pluto.

Morris, L. (1998) 'Legitimate membership of the welfare community', in Langan, M. (ed.) (1998) *Welfare: Needs, Rights and Risks,* London, Routledge in association with The Open University.

Pahl, R. (1995) 'Friendly society', *New Statesman and Society*, 10 March, pp.20–2.

Pascall, G. (1993) 'Citizenship – a feminist analysis', in Drover, G. and Kerans, P. (eds) *New Approaches to Welfare Theory*, Aldershot, Adward Elgar.

Phillips, M. (1996) *All Must Have Prizes*, London, Little, Brown and Company.

Rhodes, R. (1997) *Understanding Governance*, Buckingham, Open University Press.

Rustin, M. (1997) 'Editorial: what next?', *Soundings: The Next Ten Years,* special edition, pp.7–18.

Smith, J. (1997) 'The ideology of "family and community": New Labour abandons the welfare state', in Panitch, L. (ed.) *Socialist Register*, Suffolk, Merlin Press.

Weeks, J. (1996) 'The idea of a sexual community', *Soundings*, issue 2, pp.71–84.

Williams, F. (1989) *Critical Social Policy*, Cambridge, Polity.

Acknowledgements

Grateful acknowledgement is made to the following sources for permission to reproduce material in this book:

Text

Chapter 1: Williamson, J. (1986) *Consuming Passions, The Dynamics of Popular Culture*, Marion Boyars Publishers; Department of Health, *The Patient's Charter and You*. © Crown Copyright is reproduced with the permission of the Controller of Her Majesty's Stationery Office; Department of Education and Science, *The Parent's Charter, You and Your Child's Education*. © Crown Copyright is reproduced with the permission of the Controller of Her Majesty's Stationery Office; HMSO, *The Citizen's Charter*. © Crown Copyright is reproduced with the permission of the Controller of Her Majesty's Stationery Office; Pollitt, C. (1994) 'The Citizen's Charter: a preliminary analysis', *Public Money and Management*, April–June 1994, Blackwell Publishers, © CIPFA, 1994; Gewirtz, S., Ball, S.J. and Bowe, R. (1995) *Markets, Choice and Equity in Education*, Open University Press; Baldock, J. and Ungerson, C. (1996) 'Becoming a consumer of care: developing a sociological account of the "new community care"', in Edgell, S., Hetherington, K. and Warde, A. (eds) *Consumption Matters, The Production and Experience of Consumption*, Blackwell Publishers. Copyright © The Editorial Board of the Sociological Review, 1996; Corrigan, P. (1996) *Recreating the Public: A Responsibility for Local Government*, Lecture to the Student Centre, University of North London, 11 March 1996; **Chapter 2:** McVicar, E. (1990) *One Singer, One Song – Songs of Glasgow Folk*, Glasgow City Libraries; Hall, S. (1994) 'Basic instinct off target', *The Guardian*, © Guardian Newspapers Ltd, 1994; Pahl, R. (1995) 'Friendly society', *New Statesman and Society*, 10 March 1995, © Guardian Newspapers Ltd, 1995; Weeks, J. (1996) 'The idea of a sexual community', *Soundings*, issue 2, Spring 1996, Soundings Ltd; **Chapter 3:** Marshall, T.H. (1996) 'Citizenship and social class', in Marshall, T.H. and Bottomore, T. (eds) *Citizenship and Social Class*, Pluto; HMSO (1990) *Encouraging Citizenship, Report of the Commission on Citizenship*. © Crown Copyright is reproduced with the permission of the Controller of Her Majesty's Stationery Office; Purdy, D. (1994) 'Citizenship, basic income and the state', *New Left Review*, 208, Verso; Pascall, G. (1993) 'Citizenship – a feminist analysis', in Drover, G. and Kerans, P. (eds) *New Approaches to Welfare Theory*, Edward Elgar; Blitz, J. (1998) 'Bavaria attacks Italy over Kurdish influx', *Financial Times*, 8 January 1998.

Photographs/Illustrations

Cover: photograph by Gary Kirkham; *p.25:* Roger Beale/Financial Times; *p.43:* © Meadowhall Centre, Sheffield; *p.51:* © Guardian Newspapers Ltd; *p.61:* Port Sunlight Heritage Centre; *p.65:* Oscar Marzaroli; *p.71:* Peter Dunn, The Art of Change; *p.76:* David Simonds/New Statesman; *p.78:* Eve Arnold/Magnum; *p.82:* Hulton Getty; *p.91:* John Voos/The Independent; *p.111:* Harlow District Council; *p.115:* Format Photographers/Ulrike Preuss; *p.128:* Format Photographers/ Brenda Prince; *p.134:* courtesy of Highgate Primary School; *p.142:* Associated Sports Photography/George Herringshaw.

Table

Table 3.2: adapted from Guild, E. (1996) 'The legal framework of citizenship of the European Union', in Cesarani, D. and Fulbrook, M. (eds) *Citizenship, Nationality and Migration in Europe*, Routledge.

Index

The Open University Course Team

The Open University

Sally Baker	*Liaison Librarian/Picture Researcher*
Melanie Bayley	*Editor*
David Calderwood	*Project Controller*
Hilary Canneaux	*Course Manager*
John Clarke	*Author/Course Team Chair*
Allan Cochrane	*Author*
Lene Connolly	*Print Buying Controller*
Troy Cooper	*Author*
Nigel Draper	*Editor*
Ross Fergusson	*Author*
Sharon Gewirtz	*Reading Member*
Fiona Harris	*Editor*
Rich Hoyle	*Graphic Designer*
Gordon Hughes	*Author and Editor, Books 4 and 5*
Jonathan Hunt	*Co-publishing Co-ordinator*
Kate Hunter	*Editor*
Maggie Hutchinson	*Reading Member*
Sue Lacey	*Secretary*
Mary Langan	*Author and Editor, Book 3*
Patti Langton	*Producer, BBC/OUPC*
Helen Lentell	*Author*
Gail Lewis	*Author and Editor, Books 2 and 4*
Vic Lockwood	*Producer, BBC/OUPC*
Lilian McCoy	*Author*
Eugene McLaughlin	*Author*
Tara Marshall	*Print Buying Co-ordinator*
John Muncie	*Author/Co-Course Team Chair*
Pam Owen	*Graphic Artist*
Doreen Pendlebury	*Secretary*
Sharon Pinkney	*Author*
Michael Pryke	*Author*
Esther Saraga	*Author and Editor, Book 1*
Paul Smith	*Liaison Librarian/Picture Researcher*
Pauline Turner	*Course and Discipline Secretary*

External Contributors

Marian Barnes	*Author, Department of Social Policy and Social Work, University of Birmingham*
Janet English	*Tutor Panel, Region 11, The Open University*
Ian Gazeley	*Author, School of Social Sciences, University of Sussex*
Catherine Hall	*Author, Department of Sociology, University of Essex*
Mary J. Hickman	*Author, Irish Studies Centre, University of North London*
Eluned Jeffries	*Tutor Panel, Region 02, The Open University*
Chris Jones	*External Assessor, Professor of Social Work, University of Liverpool*
Gerry Mooney	*Author, Department of Applied Social Studies, University of Paisley*
Lydia Morris	*Author, Department of Sociology, University of Essex*
Janet Newman	*Author, School of Public Policy, University of Birmingham*
Lynne Poole	*Tutor Panel, Region 11, The Open University*
Pat Thane	*Author, School of Social Sciences, University of Sussex*